LECTURE NOTES ON
RESPIRATORY DISEASE

LECTURE NOTES ON
RESPIRATORY DISEASE

WRITTEN AND ILLUSTRATED BY

R. A. L. BREWIS

MD, FRCP

Senior Lecturer in Medicine,
University of Newcastle upon Tyne
Consultant Physician,
Royal Victoria Infirmary,
Newcastle upon Tyne

FOURTH PRINTING

BLACKWELL SCIENTIFIC PUBLICATIONS

OXFORD LONDON EDINBURGH MELBOURNE

© 1975 Blackwell Scientific Publications
Osney Mead, Oxford OX2 0EL
8 John Street, London WC1N 2ES
9 Forrest Road, Edinburgh, EH1 2QH
P.O. Box 9, North Balwyn, Victoria, Australia.

ISBN 0 632 00651 X

First published 1975

Revised reprint 1976
Reprinted 1977, 1978

Printed in Great Britain by
Billing & Sons Limited,
Guildford, London and Worcester

CONTENTS

PREFACE

The aim of this book is to present a concise review of respiratory disease. In addition to offering the medical student an alternative to attending lectures it is hoped that this book might provide the MRCP candidate with his basic minimum requirements in the respiratory field and the more mature general medical reader with a painless refresher course.

The emphasis throughout is on information which is useful and relevant to everyday clinical medicine. In reviewing pulmonary physiology and the assessment of pulmonary function all unnecessary complexities, symbols and equations have been avoided and attention has been focused on concepts and investigations which are in everyday use. A number of rare conditions receive little or no mention but the practical aspects of management of the commoner disorders are dealt with in some detail.

Numerous teachers, colleagues, students and patients have played a part in the development of my interest in respiratory disease but I owe a particular debt to Professor Jack Howell for opening my eyes to some of the special fascinations of the subject. I am grateful to Miss Veronica Downey for help with typing; without her watchful eye on my other commitments it would have been impossible to attend to the business of writing. I am grateful to Dr Martin Farebrother for reading parts of the manuscript and to Mr Per Saugman for his encouragement and courtesy. I hope to express my gratitude to my wife and family by seeing a little more of them.

R.A.L.B.

Newcastle upon Tyne, 1974

CHAPTER 1 · REVIEW OF ANATOMY OF THE LUNG

Surface anatomy

The position of the lungs and some useful external landmarks are indicated in Fig. 1.1. A few points are worthy of special mention:
1 The apices of the lungs extend well above the clavicles.
2 The posterior surface of the lungs extends further downwards than the anterior surface.
3 The upper lobes are situated *in front of* the lower lobes so that the lung immediately below the anterior chest wall is largely derived from the upper lobe and that beneath the posterior chest wall is mainly lower lobe.

Subdivisions of the lung

The lungs are divided into **lobes**—three on the right and two on the left—which are separated by slit-like invaginations of the pleural space. Each lobe has its own lobar bronchus. Each lobe is further subdivided by incomplete fibrous septa which extend inwards from the pleural surface into **bronchopulmonary segments**. Each bronchopulmonary segment is supplied by its own segmental bronchus and the usual arrangement of the segmental bronchi is shown in Fig. 1.2. Some pathological processes may be limited to particular segments which may be identified radiologically. Smaller incomplete fibrous septa are present within each segment which outline individual **lobules**. Lobules are about 1 cm in diameter and of variable shape but generally they are pyramidal with the apex towards the bronchiole which supplies them. The anatomy of the lobule is illustrated in Fig. 1.3. Each lobule contains 3 to 5 **acini**, each supplied by a terminal bronchiole. Acini are sometimes visualised on the chest X-ray when they are filled with secretions or bronchographic contrast medium producing a blotchy appearance sometimes referred to as acinar pattern.

Branching of the airways

The trachea divides into two main bronchi. The left main bronchus is longer than the right and comes off at a more abrupt angle. The right main bronchus is more directly in line with the trachea so that inhaled material tends to enter the right lung more readily than the left. The main bronchi

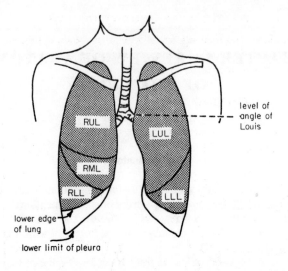

(a)

(b)

Fig. 1.1. *Surface anatomy.* (a) Anterior view of the lungs. (b) Lateral view of right side of chest at resting end-expiratory position. RUL: right upper lobe; RML: right middle lobe; RLL: right lower lobe; LUL: left upper lobe; LLL: left lower lobe.

divide into lobar and then segmental bronchi as shown in Fig. 1.2. Further divisions occur in an uneven dichotomous fashion; that is the branches at a division are not necessarily of the same size.

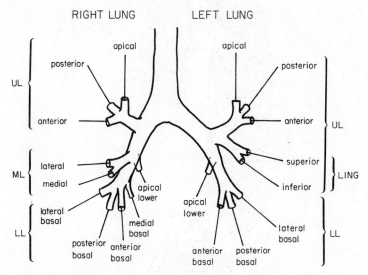

Fig. 1.2. *Diagram of bronchopulmonary segments.* UL: upper lobe; ML: middle lobe; LL: lower lobe; LING: lingula.

Bronchi

Bronchi are airways with cartilage in their walls. There are about 10 divisions of bronchi beyond the tracheal bifurcation. Smaller airways without cartilage in their walls are referred to as **bronchioles**. The term **respiratory bronchiole** refers to the peripheral bronchioles with alveoli in their walls. The bronchiole immediately proximal to the appearance of alveoli is known as the **terminal bronchiole**. The number of divisions between the bifurcation of the trachea and the terminal bronchiole varies between about 9 and 32. In general there are fewer branches to acini near the hilum and more branches to the peripherally situated acini.

Collateral ventilation

Holes in the alveolar walls known as pores of Kohn allow communication between parts of the lobule supplied by different respiratory bronchioles. There is a variable degree of communication at alveolar level between neighbouring lobules. Collateral ventilation through these communications is of importance in panacinar emphysema. In this condition they are increased in size and number as part of the parenchymal destructive process.

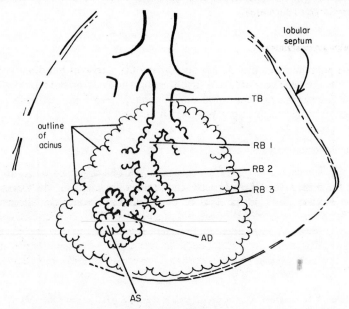

Fig. 1.3. *Diagram of the anatomy of the lobule.*
The lobule lies within incomplete fibrous septa and contains several acini. The borders of individual acini are not normally discernible. Each acinus is supplied by a terminal bronchiole (TB). There are about three orders of respiratory bronchioles with alveoli in their walls (RB1, RB2, RB3) which lead to alveolar ducts (AD) which are formed from the mouths of alveoli and alveolar sacs (AS).

Pulmonary vasculature

Pulmonary artery

The pulmonary artery divides into left and right pulmonary arteries which provide branches accompanying the branches of the bronchial tree. The arteries accompanying bronchi are elastic but have only thin muscular coats. The arteries accompanying bronchioles have well-developed medial muscular coats which become thinner peripherally. The **arterioles** accompanying terminal and respiratory bronchioles are thin walled and contain little smooth muscle.

Capillary network

The capillary network in the alveolar walls is very dense and provides a very large surface area.

Pulmonary venules

The pulmonary venules do not accompany the arterioles but drain laterally to the periphery of lobules and then pass centrally in the interlobular and intersegmental septa ultimately joining to form the four main pulmonary veins which empty into the left atrium.

The bronchial circulation

Small bronchial arteries usually arise from the descending aorta and travel in the outer layers of the bronchi and bronchioles supplying the tissues of the airways down to the level of the respiratory bronchiole. Bronchial veins drain into radicles of the pulmonary vein. They thus contribute a small amount of desaturated blood which accounts for part of the 'physiological shunt' observed in normal individuals. The bronchial arteries may be much enlarged in some diseases (e.g. severe bronchiectasis, pulmonary fibrosis).

Structure of the airways

Trachea

The trachea has cartilaginous horseshoe-shaped 'rings' supporting anterior and lateral walls. The posterior wall is flaccid and during coughing, when intrathoracic pressure is raised and the glottis opens, this soft posterior segment billows forwards reducing the lumen of the trachea to a U-shaped slit. This results in a high linear velocity of air-flow which produces a shearing effect which hastens the clearance of any excess of secretions. The trachea is lined with ciliated epithelium which contains goblet cells.

Bronchi

The bronchi have irregular plates of cartilage in their walls. Smooth muscle is arranged in spiral fashion internal to the cartilaginous plates and attached to them. The muscle coat becomes more complete distally as the cartilaginous plates become more fragmentary.

The epithelial lining is ciliated and includes goblet cells which become less numerous peripherally. Larger bronchi also have acinar mucus-secreting glands in the sub-mucosa. Hypertrophy of these glands is one of the more striking features of chronic bronchitis.

Bronchioles

The bronchioles have no cartilage in their walls. The muscular layer becomes progressively thinner peripherally but some strands of smooth muscle persist to the level of respiratory bronchioles and possibly beyond. The epithelium is made up of a single layer of ciliated cells with only very occasional goblet cells. A granulated cell known as the Clara cell appears in the wall of distal bronchioles and this cell is suspected of possessing secretory properties. It may contribute mucus to alveolar fluid making up the foundation of the mucous blanket which is propelled upwards by ciliary action.

Ciliated epithelium

Ciliated epithelial cells possess about 200 cilia each 3 to 6 μ in length. Cilia beat with a whip-like action very rapidly (the beat frequency is probably of the order of 1,000 per minute). Organised waves of contraction pass regularly from cell to cell. The cilia beat in a layer of thin fluid beneath a more viscous layer of mucus. The mucous sheet is about 5 μ thick and carries a load of macrophages, cellular debris, inhaled particles etc. In the trachea the mucous sheet moves upwards at about 1·5 cm per minute. Ciliary action is impaired by drying of the secretions, increase in thickness of the mucous sheet and by inhaled noxious agents such as cigarette smoke.

Alveolar structure

Alveoli are about 0·1 to 0·2 mm in diameter and take up a variety of shapes depending on the arrangement of adjacent alveoli. The structure of the alveolar wall is represented diagrammatically in Fig. 1.4. The capillaries are completely lined by flattened endothelial cells resting on a complete basement membrane. The alveoli are completely lined by a layer of alveolar cells which are of two types.

Type I pneumocyte

These cells have extensive flattened processes which extend to cover most of the internal surface of the alveoli. Only the nuclei of these cells are evident on light microscopy.

Type II pneumocyte

These cells are less numerous and more globular than the type I pneumocytes. Electron microscopy reveals that these cells contain bodies with a concentric lamellated structure. There is evidence which suggests that these bodies are concerned with the manufacture or storage of surfactant (p. 27).

Alveoli contain phagocytic macrophages (p. 215).

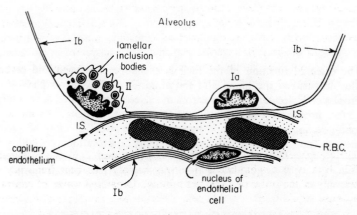

Fig. 1.4. Diagram of structure of alveolar wall as revealed by electron microscopy. Ia Type I pneumocyte; Ib Flattened extension of Type I pneumocyte covering most of the internal surface of the alveolus. II Type II pneumocyte with lamellar inclusion bodies which are probably the site of surfactant formation. I.S. Interstitial space. R.B.C. Red blood corpuscle. Pneumocytes and endothelial cells rest upon thin continuous basement membranes which are not shown.

Interstitial space

There is a potential space between the alveolar cells and the capillary basement membrane which is only apparent in disease states. It is continuous with the interstitial space surrounding bronchi and blood vessels (p. 193).

Lymphatic vessels

Lymphatic channels are present in the interstitial space. They accompany the bronchial tree at least as far as the level of the respiratory bronchioles and supply the walls of the airway as well as the pulmonary interstitium. Lymphatics are also found in the interlobular septa and are abundant beneath the pleural surface. Drainage of lymph is towards the intrapulmonary lymph nodes adjacent to the proximal bronchi and thereafter to the mediastinal lymph nodes.

CHAPTER 2 · REVIEW OF RESPIRATORY PHYSIOLOGY

The essential function of the lung is exchange of oxygen and carbon dioxide between the blood and the atmosphere. This takes place by a process of molecular diffusion across the alveolar membrane. A very large surface area is necessary to achieve this gaseous exchange—in an adult man it is estimated that the surface area of the alveoli is about 60 square metres. The structure of the lung represents an evolutionary solution to the problems of accommodating this huge membrane, moving air and blood to and from its surfaces and protecting it from external insults.

MECHANICAL CONSIDERATIONS

Breathing

Inspiration is brought about by descent of the diaphragm and movement of the ribs upwards and outwards under the influence of the external intercostal muscles. Expiration is the consequence of gradually lessening contraction of the intercostal muscles allowing the lungs to collapse under the influence of their own elastic forces. This pattern of breathing—active inspiratory muscle contraction and passive expiration—is that normally encountered in quiet breathing at rest but other mechanisms are involved in other breathing patterns. In particular abdominal muscle contraction is brought into play during very rapid breathing and in breathing out to a position of full expiration (residual volume).

Lung compliance

The inherent elastic property of the lungs causes them to tend to retract from the chest wall causing a negative intrapleural pressure. The strength of the retractive force is related to the degree of stretching of the lung tissue—that is to lung volume. At high lung volumes the intrapleural pressure is more negative than at low lung volumes. The term lung compliance refers to the relationship between this retractive force and lung volume. Lung compliance is expressed as **the change in lung volume brought about by unit change in transpulmonary (intrapleural) pressure** and the units employed are litres per kilopascal or litres per cm of water. Fig. 2.1 shows

8

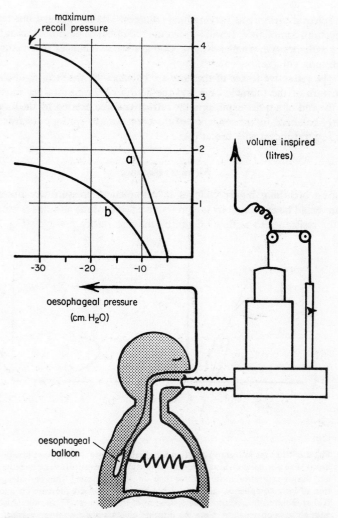

Fig. 2.1. *Lung compliance.* Oesophageal pressure is noted at a number of different volumes (each held momentarily with glottis open). The relationship between transpulmonary pressure and volume of air inspired is plotted for 2 individuals a and b. Lung compliance is an expression of the change in lung volume which accompanied unit change in transpulmonary pressure. In the case of a, lung compliance is normal (= 0·25 1/cm H_2O approx. or 2·5 l.kPa^{-1}). In the case of b, a smaller change in volume accompanies each unit change in pressure and compliance is low (= 0·1 1/cm H_2O approx. or 1·0 l.kPa^{-1}). Note that lung compliance becomes progressively less as lung volume increases.

intrapleural pressure at varying lung volumes. The slope of the line represents lung compliance. It will be seen that compliance becomes less at high lung volumes (i.e. smaller volume changes follow changes in pressure at high lung volume).

The retractive forces of the lung are balanced by the semi-rigid elastic structure of the thoracic cage and the action of the respiratory muscles. At the end of a quiet expiration the retractive force exerted by the lungs is nicely balanced by the tendency of the chest wall to spring outwards and the respiratory muscles are at rest.

Airways resistance

During breathing bigger changes in intrapleural pressure are observed than would be explained by lung retractive forces alone and this is because of the resistance to airflow offered by the respiratory passages (Fig. 2.2).

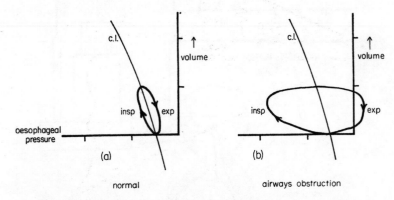

Fig. 2.2. Changes in intrapleural (oesophageal) pressure during quiet breathing. (a) in a normal individual. During inspiration the pressure is more negative and during expiration more positive than would be expected from consideration of lung compliance. c.l.: compliance line. The excessive pressure change is that required to overcome the resistance of the airways. (b) an individual with airways obstruction. Here the pressure changes are even more marked. During expiration oesophageal pressure is actually above atmospheric indicating compression of the lungs by expiratory musculature.

The additional pressure change depends upon the calibre of the airways and also upon the rate of airflow. The greater part of the total airways resistance is situated in the large airways—main bronchi, trachea and larynx—but in disease the increase in resistance generally involves the much smaller distal airways. The airways behave differently during inspiration and expiration. During inspiration pulmonary elastic recoil causes the

airways to open. During expiration the pull on the walls of the airways
diminishes so that there is an increasing tendency towards closure of the
airways.

The flow-limiting mechanism

Consider the model of the lung described in Fig. 2.3. During expiration the
resistance of the distal airway (Res) will cause a drop in pressure between
a and b so that the floppy segment will tend to collapse. It will be protected

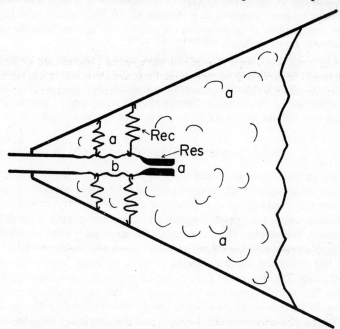

Fig. 2.3. Diagram of a model of the lung to demonstrate the flow-limiting
mechanism (see text). The chest is represented as a bellows. The airways of the
lungs are represented collectively as having a distal resistive segment (Res) and
a more proximal collapsible or 'floppy' segment. The walls of the floppy segment are kept apart by the retractive force of lung recoil (Rec).

from collapse by the retractive force of the surrounding lung parenchyma
(Rec). The extent of the pressure drop from a to b is proportional to the
rate of air-flow. There will be a critical rate of air-flow which results in b
being so much lower than a that the retractive force of the lung is overcome and the floppy segment closes. The closure limits the air-flow leading
to less dramatic pressure drop from a to b which permits some re-opening
of the floppy segment. It will be apparent that the system will control the

maximum rate of air-flow to a level determined by lung recoil (assuming
that the resistance of the upstream segment (Res) remains constant). Lung
recoil depends upon how stretched the lungs are and it should now be
clear why high expiratory flow rates are obtainable at high lung volumes,
but as lung volume decreases during expiration the maximum flow rate
becomes progressively less and less. For each lung volume there is a particular maximum flow rate which cannot be exceeded no matter how great
the expiratory effort.

The shape of the forced expiratory spirogram (Fig. 6.4) is thus determined by inherent mechanical properties of the lung and is to a large
extent independent of effort above a certain level. This explains its very
remarkable reproducibility.

When airways resistance is increased in disease a much greater pressure-
drop occurs between a and b so that the supporting effect of recoil pressure
(Rec) tends to be overcome at more modest rates of expiratory air-flow than
in the normal. In this situation there is obvious advantage in breathing at
a high lung volume which results in a greater lung recoil (Rec).

Where does the air go?

During an inspiration the distribution of air within the lungs is uneven
because the compliance of different parts of the lungs is not uniform and
because the resistance of the airways is also uneven. One of the most
obvious causes of the uneven distribution of lung compliance is the effect
of gravity. The weight of the lungs causes the upper parts to be kept under
a greater stretch than the more dependent zones and the upper parts are
thus less compliant. During inspiration more air tends to pass into the
lower zones. The uppermost parts of the lungs may be regarded as already
almost fully stretched and thus less 'receptive'. The analogy of a suspended
spring may help to make the effect of gravity clearer (Fig. 2.4). The greater
ventilation of the lower zones during quiet breathing is not inappropriate
because gravity also directs pulmonary blood flow preferentially to the
lower zones.

Unevenness of ventilation is also present within the lungs on a more
miniature scale—adjacent lobules and even adjacent alveoli may have
different compliances and, in response to a change of intrapleural pressure,
may accept more or less air than expected. Local differences of airways
resistance will also cause some unevenness in the distribution of inspired
air. The effect of an increase in airways resistance is to reduce the rate of
air-flow produced by a given change in intrapleural pressure—that is to
delay filling of the lung or part of the lung. During extremely slow breathing the effect of increased airways resistance will be very small and air
will pass into the most receptive (most compliant) parts of the lungs. But
when breathing is more rapid, local increase in airways resistance will

hamper the acceptance of air by the part of the lung in question because there may be insufficient time for proper filling of the region.

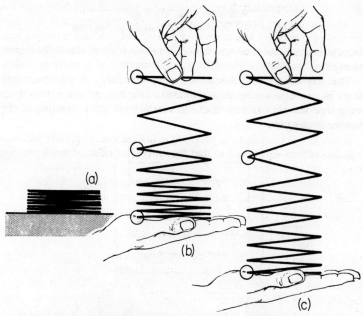

Fig. 2.4. *Gravity and regional ventilation*

The 'Slinky' spring used to demonstrate greater ventilation of the bases in the normal upright lung. (a) The 'Slinky' spring in its resting condition. (b) The spring extended upwards to represent the normal lung suspended within the pleural cavity in a stretched condition by the effect of atmospheric pressure. The circles mark the top, middle and bottom of the spring (lung) under these conditions. (c) The bottom hand has been lowered to represent inspiration. Most of the increase in length has been contributed by the lower part of the spring; the upper part was already at almost full stretch before 'inspiration'. In the lung the upper zones are relatively more stretched than the lower zones and their compliance is thus less. During inspiration under such conditions more air goes to the bases. This is appropriate since the bases are relatively better perfused than the upper zones.

The 'Slinky' spring also permits exploration of the effects of gravity in abnormal lungs. 1. When lung volume is progressively reduced it is evident that collapse is much more likely to occur in the lower zones. 2. Lung recoil is evidently lower in the lower zones so that the smaller airways are not held open so forcibly. In the presence of diffuse airways obstruction the obstruction tends to be more severe in the lower zones. Many airways in the lower zones close on expiration and ventilation is directed more to the upper zones.

The local differences referred to are probably small in the healthy lung as the network of the lung parenchyma distributes forces fairly evenly but

local differences become important in disease of the lung parenchyma
which tends to be patchy in distribution.

Where does the blood go?
(haemodynamics of the pulmonary circulation)

The pulmonary circulation normally offers a much lower resistance to perfusion than the systemic circulation and it operates at a lower perfusion
pressure. The difference between the mean pulmonary artery pressure and
left atrial pressure in the resting individual is only of the order of 15
mmHg—or less than one-sixth of the effective perfusion pressure of the
systemic circulation.

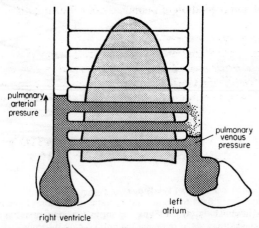

Fig. 2.5. *Model of the pulmonary circulation.*
At rest in the erect position the bulk of the cardiac output passes through the
bases and the apices are virtually unperfused because pulmonary artery
pressure is not sufficiently high. If pulmonary artery pressure rises because of
increased cardiac output, increased pulmonary vascular resistance or increased
pulmonary venous pressure then more of the pulmonary circulation will be
filled.

At rest in the erect position gravity exerts a major effect upon the
distribution of blood within the lungs. Blood passes predominantly to the
bases and there is barely any perfusion of the apices—the pulmonary
circulation is not 'full' (Fig. 2.5). If pulmonary artery pressure rises either
through an increase in pulmonary vascular resistance or an increase in
cardiac output then more of the pulmonary circulation in the upper zones
is brought into play.

An increase in left atrial pressure secondary to left-sided cardiac
disease will dam back blood in the lungs raising pulmonary venous pressure

so that veins further up the lungs become filled. Pulmonary artery pressure must increase if the circulation is to be maintained so that more of the circulation in the upper zones is opened up.

In addition to the major regional effect of gravity there are other factors which affect the distribution of blood within the lungs and these may be quite localised.

1. HYPOXIA

Hypoxia is a potent pulmonary vasoconstrictor. The response seems to be a direct response of arterial smooth muscle to low oxygen tension in the lung surrounding it. By this means blood tends to be diverted away from underventilated areas of the lungs—a process which may be looked upon as a form of autoregulation of pulmonary blood distribution.

2. ALVEOLAR PRESSURE

The pulmonary capillaries are capable of being compressed as they pass through the alveolar walls if alveolar pressure rises above capillary pressure. Under certain circumstances local increases in alveolar pressure may develop and have an effect upon the distribution of blood flow.

GAS EXCHANGE AND VENTILATION/ PERFUSION RELATIONSHIPS

Overall gas exchange

During steady-state conditions the relationship between the amount of CO_2 produced by the body and the amount of oxygen absorbed depends upon the metabolic activity of the body as a whole and is referred to as the Respiratory Quotient (R.Q. or R).

$$R.Q. = \frac{CO_2 \text{ produced}}{O_2 \text{ absorbed}}$$

The actual value is dependent upon the principal metabolic substrate of the body at the time. R.Q. varies from about 0·7 during pure fat metabolism to 1·0 during pure carbohydrate metabolism and is usually found to be about 0·8 at rest during the day. Overall R.Q. is important but consideration of gas exchange in the lung is made much easier if its value is assumed to be 1·0. Oxygen and CO_2 are exchanged in equal amounts in this situation.

Alveolar ventilation

It is obvious that not all of the air drawn into the lungs reaches the alveoli. The volume of air filling the airways down to the level of the terminal bronchiole at the end of an inspiration is termed the anatomical dead-space. It is less obvious that even in the normal lung not all of the inspired air which actually reaches the alveoli participates evenly in gas exchange. Some alveoli are relatively overventilated and some are underventilated relative to the blood flow they receive. To overcome the difficulties of analysing such a complicated state of affairs the expired air can be regarded as being derived from two hypothetical sources; 1, ideal alveoli all of which contain alveolar air with the same P_{CO_2} as arterial blood and 2, other areas of lung which do not participate in gas exchange at all. These two components of the total ventilation are termed alveolar ventilation and deadspace ventilation. Alveolar ventilation is effective ventilation. Deadspace ventilation is ineffective ventilation. Deadspace ventilation is normally less than a quarter of the total but the proportion varies with breathing frequency, exercise and other influences.

Effect of changing alveolar ventilation

For the moment discussion will be limited to the situation which exists in an idealised normal lung in which all of the units have well-matched ventilation and perfusion and all behave identically.

CARBON DIOXIDE

If CO_2 is being produced by the tissues of the body at a constant rate the P_{CO_2} of alveolar air depends only upon the amount of outside air that the CO_2 is mixed with in the alveoli; that is the P_{CO_2} depends only upon alveolar ventilation. If alveolar ventilation is high, the P_{CO_2} will be low; if alveolar ventilation falls, the P_{CO_2} will rise. Alveolar P_{CO_2} is inversely proportional to alveolar ventilation.

OXYGEN

The level of alveolar P_{O_2} also varies with alveolar ventilation. If alveolar ventilation is greatly increased the steady uptake of oxygen by the body will only slightly reduce the alveolar P_{O_2} below the level in the outside air. On the other hand if alveolar ventilation is very low then the alveolar P_{O_2} will fall to a low level. Alveolar (or arterial) P_{O_2} varies directly with alveolar ventilation. Measurement of arterial P_{O_2} is less reliable than measurement of P_{CO_2} as an index of alveolar ventilation because it is profoundly affected by regional changes in ventilation-perfusion ratio as will be shown below.

Measurement of alveolar or arterial P_{CO_2} is the only reliable guide to the adequacy of alveolar ventilation.

The changes in alveolar ventilation just described are examples of changes in the ventilation-perfusion ratio (V/Q) of the lungs as a whole.

EFFECT OF OVERALL INCREASE IN V/Q

If alveolar ventilation increases in relation to perfusion then alveolar P_{CO_2} will fall and alveolar P_{O_2} will rise.

EFFECT OF OVERALL FALL IN V/Q

If alveolar ventilation falls in relation to perfusion alveolar P_{CO_2} will rise and alveolar P_{O_2} will fall.

In the model under discussion all of the alveoli behave identically and the arterial blood therefore shows the same changes in P_{CO_2} and P_{O_2} as the alveolar air.

RELATIONSHIP BETWEEN P_{CO_2} AND P_{O_2}

The possible combinations of P_{CO_2} and P_{O_2} can be explored with the help

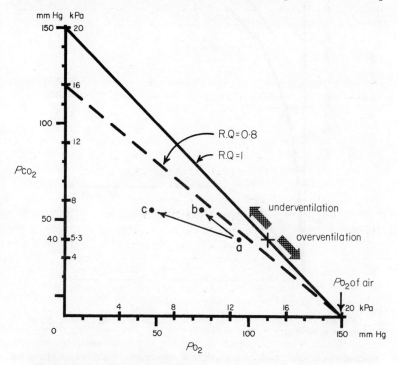

Fig. 2.6. *Oxygen-Carbon dioxide diagram*
The continuous and interrupted lines describe the possible combinations of P_{CO_2} and P_{O_2} in alveolar air when the R.Q. is 1·0 and 0·8 respectively. (a) A hypothetical sample of arterial blood. (b) Progressive underventilation. (c) P_{O_2} lower than can be accounted for by underventilation alone.

of the diagram shown in Fig. 2.6. Moist atmospheric air at 37°C has a P_{O_2} of about 20 kPa (150 mmHg). In our model oxygen could be exchanged with CO_2 in the alveoli to produce any combination of Po_2 and Pco_2 described by the oblique line which joins Po_2 20 kPa (150 mmHg) and Pco_2 20 kPa (150 mmHg). The position of the cross on this line represents the composition of a hypothetical sample of alveolar air. A fall in alveolar

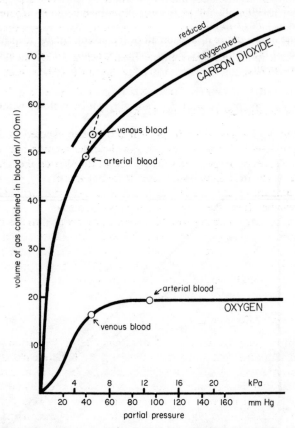

Fig. 2.7. The oxygen and carbon dioxide dissociation curves of blood drawn to the same scale.

ventilation would result in an upwards movement of this point along the line and conversely an increase in alveolar ventilation would result in a downward movement of the point.

In practice the R.Q. is rarely 1·0 and it is nearer the truth to say;

$$\text{Alveolar } Po_2 + (\text{alveolar } Pco_2/\text{R.Q.}) = 20 \text{ kPa (150 mmHg)}.$$

The interrupted oblique line represents the combinations of Pco_2 and Po_2 encountered when the R.Q. is 0·8. Point *a* represents the Pco_2 and Po_2

of arterial blood (it lies a little to the left of the R.Q. 0·8 line because of the small normal alveolar-arterial oxygen tension difference). Point b represents the arterial gas tensions after a period of underventilation.

This relationship between P_{CO_2} and P_{O_2} is very useful clinically. For example, if the arterial P_{CO_2} and P_{O_2} were those represented by point c it would be clear that the fall in P_{O_2} was more than could be accounted for on the grounds of reduced alveolar ventilation. An appreciation of the relationship between P_{CO_2} and P_{O_2} provides some safeguard against certain errors in blood gas measurement. Even when the R.Q. is 1·0 the sum of P_{CO_2} and P_{O_2} should not exceed 20 kPa (150 mmHg) when breathing air.

Review of the carriage of CO_2 and O_2 by blood

The quantity of a gas which blood will carry when exposed to different partial pressures of the gas is described by the dissociation curve. The dissociation curves of oxygen and CO_2 are shown together on the same scale in Fig. 2.7. The most important points to be noted are:

1   The amount of CO_2 carried by blood is roughly proportional to the P_{CO_2} prevailing (over the range normally encountered).

2   The quantity of oxygen carried is roughly proportional to the P_{O_2} only over a very limited range—from about 2·7 to 6·7 kPa (20 to 50 mmHg.)

3   Above this level there is less additional oxygen carried with each increase in P_{O_2} and above 13·3 kPa (100 mmHg) the haemoglobin is fully saturated and hardly any additional oxygen is carried.

Effect of local differences in V/Q

In the normal lung the vast majority of alveoli receive ventilation and perfusion in about the right proportion (a in Fig. 2.8). In diffuse disease of the lung, however, it is usual for ventilation and perfusion to be irregularly distributed so that a greater scatter of V/Q ratios is encountered (b in Fig. 2.8). Even if the *overall* V/Q remains normal there is wide local variation in V/Q. Looking at Fig. 2.8 it is tempting to suppose that the effects of the alveoli with low V/Q might be nicely balanced by the alveoli with high V/Q. In fact this is not the case; the increased range of V/Q within the lung affects the transport of CO_2 and O_2 differently.

In Fig. 2.9, b and c are regions of low and high V/Q respectively and the result of mixing blood from these two regions is shown at d where arterial CO_2 and O_2 content are represented.

EFFECT UPON ARTERIAL CO_2 CONTENT
Blood with a high CO_2 content returning from low V/Q areas mixes with blood with a low CO_2 content returning from high V/Q areas and the net

CO_2 content of arterial blood may be nearly normal as the two balance out.

EFFECT UPON ARTERIAL O_2 CONTENT

Here the situation is different. Blood returning from low V/Q areas has a low Po_2 and a low O_2 content but there is a limit to which this deficit can

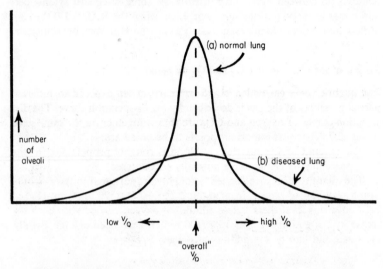

Fig. 2.8. Distribution of Ventilation/Perfusion relationships within the lungs. Although the overall ventilation/perfusion (V/Q) ratio is the same in the two examples shown, the increased spread of V/Q ratios within the diseased lung (b) will result in a lower arterial oxygen tension and content than in the normal lung (a). Arterial Pco_2 will be similar in the two situations shown.

be made good by mixture with blood returning from high V/Q areas which, although it has a high Po_2, cannot carry more than the 'normal' quantity of oxygen as its O_2 content is limited by saturation of the haemoglobin.

1   Areas of low V/Q result in a rise in arterial CO_2 content and a fall in arterial O_2 content.

2   Increased ventilation of areas of high V/Q may balance the effect upon CO_2 content but will only partly correct the reduction in O_2 content of arterial blood; a degree of hypoxaemia is inevitable.

3   It follows that where arterial oxygen levels are lower than would be expected from consideration of the Pco_2 there are probably local areas of low V/Q present in the lungs.

VENTILATION /
PERFUSION
RATIO

DISSOCIATION
CURVE

BLOOD GAS
CONTENT

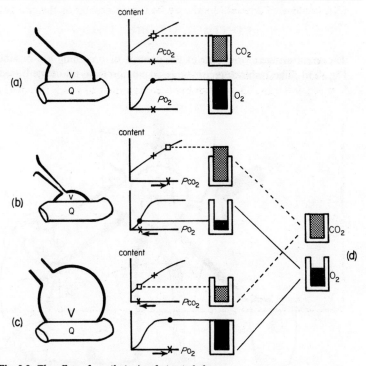

Fig. 2.9. *The effect of ventilation/perfusion imbalance*

(a) **Appropriate V/Q.** The ventilation (V)/perfusion (Q) ratio is shown diagrammatically on the left. When ventilation is appropriately matched to perfusion in an alveolus or in the lung as a whole the Pco_2 is about 40 mmHg and the Po_2 is about 95 mmHg. The dissociation curves shown in the centre of the diagram describe the relationship between the blood gas tension and the amount of gas carried by the blood. The normal blood gas contents are represented very diagrammatically on the right.

(b) **Low V/Q.** Reduced ventilation relative to blood flow results in a rise in Pco_2 and a fall in Po_2. Reference to the dissociation curves shows that this produces a rise in arterial CO_2 content and a fall in oxygen content.

(c) **High V/Q.** Increased ventilation relative to blood flow results in a fall in Pco_2 and a rise in Po_2. Reference to the dissociation curves shows that this results in a fall in CO_2 content below the normal level but in the case of oxygen there is no increase in content above the normal level.

In health the vast majority of alveoli have an appropriate balance of ventilation and perfusion and the arterial blood has a normal CO_2 and oxygen content as shown in a. In many disease states the V/Q ratio varies widely between areas. Such variation always results in disturbance of blood gas content. The effects of areas of low V/Q are not corrected by areas of high V/Q. The result of mixing blood from areas of low and high V/Q is shown diagrammatically on the extreme right of the diagram (d). It will be seen that with respect to CO_2 content the high content of blood from underventilated areas is balanced by the low content of blood from overventilated areas. However in the case of oxygen, the low content of blood from underventilated areas cannot be compensated for by an equivalent increase in the oxygen content of blood from overventilated areas. *Arterial hypoxaemia is inevitable if there are areas of low V/Q (relative underventilation or over-perfusion).*

CONTROL OF BREATHING

The main elements involved in the control of breathing are outlined in
Fig. 2.10. The respiratory centre is an anatomically ill-defined group of

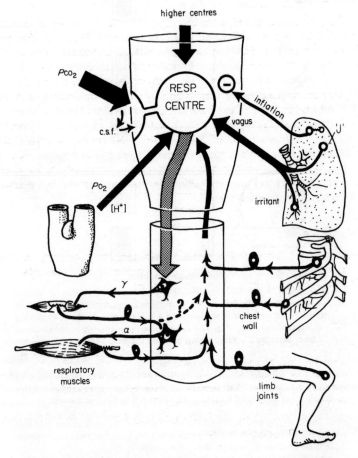

Fig. 2.10. *Control of ventilation.* Diagram showing some of the more important
factors involved (see text).

interconnected neurones which is responsible for generating phasic motor
discharges which ultimately pass by phrenic and intercostal nerves to the
respiratory musculature. The medullary discharge is integrated at spinal

level and the final output is matched to the mechanical loading of the lungs and chest through the operation of muscle spindles.

Chemical factors in the control of ventilation

Carbon dioxide

The Pco_2 of arterial blood is the most important factor in the regulation of ventilation. Normal individuals maintain an arterial Pco_2 very close to 5·3 kPa (40 mmHg) and an increase above this level provokes hyperventilation. Arterial Pco_2 exerts its effect upon the respiratory centre by stimulating sensitive areas on the surface of the medulla which are bathed by C.S.F. CO_2 may act on these sensitive areas directly and also by diffusing into the C.S.F. which has less efficient buffering properties than blood. Change in C.S.F. Pco_2 produces a greater change in [H^+] than that which occurs in blood. The C.S.F.-mediated effect is probably more potent than the direct effect and this may account for certain anomalies encountered in clinical practice. When longstanding disorders of acid base balance are corrected the ventilatory control may lag behind despite improvement in the acid-base status of the arterial blood.

Hydrogen ion [H^+]

Increase in [H^+] (fall in pH) stimulates ventilation. Pco_2 and [H^+] are able to stimulate ventilation independently. [H^+] probably exerts its influence by stimulation of the carotid and aortic bodies.

Oxygen

A fall in arterial oxygen tension stimulates ventilation. The effect of oxygen tension is very small above a Po_2 of about 8 kPa (60 mmHg). Hypoxia sensitises the respiratory centre to CO_2 and the effects of a fall in Po_2 and an increase in Pco_2 are more than merely additive. Hypoxia exerts its effects by stimulating the carotid and aortic bodies. These receptors are sensitive to reduced oxygen delivery arising from circulatory failure as well as that due to reduced arterial oxygen tension.

Neurogenic factors

1. Higher centres

Sleep and coma of whatever cause reduce the response to the normal ventilatory stimuli. Alarm and excitement tend to stimulate ventilation. Part of the ventilatory response to exercise may be initiated by higher centres as hyperventilation commonly precedes the actual start of exercise. Voluntary control can of course over-ride the normal automatic control of breathing.

2. Brain stem

Breathing is interrupted during coughing, swallowing, phonation and other semi-automatic activities. Damage to the brain stem may cause hyperventilation, hypoventilation or other disturbances of control.

3. Vagus

The vagus carries afferent stimuli from the respiratory tract which may influence breathing.

(A) INFLATION REFLEX (HERING-BREUER)

In animals stretching of the lungs causes reflex inhibition of subsequent inspiration. This effect is difficult to demonstrate in man and probably unimportant.

(B) J RECEPTORS

These are situated deep in the parenchyma of the lung and excitation stimulates ventilation. Pulmonary embolism and pulmonary oedema are among the conditions thought to excite the receptors.

(C) IRRITANT RECEPTORS

These receptors are probably situated in the distal bronchioles. Irritation and local distortion are thought to stimulate them and this results in increased ventilation. It is possible that these receptors may play a part in the production of the hyperventilation which accompanies asthma, inhalation of irritant vapours and gases, pulmonary embolism, pneumonia etc. Bronchoconstriction appears to be a part of the reflex response.

(D) COUGH RECEPTORS

The larger bronchi and the trachea possess vagally innervated receptors which are sensitive to contact and irritants. Stimulation provokes the cough reflex and a variable degree of bronchoconstriction.

4. Spinal cord

Stretch receptors in muscle tendons and joint position receptors are stimulated by chest movement and may be particularly sensitive to chest deformation caused by increased respiratory effort. The central effect of this sensory information is uncertain. Stimulation of joint receptors in the limbs enhances ventilation and this may be a contributory cause of the hyperpnoea of exercise.

5. Exercise

Ventilation increases in direct proportion to work rate during exercise. Pco_2, Po_2 and [H^+] generally remain normal and cannot explain the ventilatory response. Psychic factors and the limb joint reflex already mentioned are similarly inadequate explanations. A number of hypotheses have been suggested which explain the observed facts but no comprehensive analysis of the control of ventilation has attained general acceptance.

Respiratory sensations

An awareness of the behaviour of the lungs and of the act of breathing may be compiled from several sources. These include vision, hearing, the sensation of movement and temperature change in the upper respiratory tract, sensations originating in vagal irritant and cough receptors, and sensations of chest wall movement.

Appreciation of breath-size and resistance to breathing is probably mainly derived from muscle tendon and joint receptors in the thorax although the skin receptors may contribute some information. Muscle spindles may provide further sensory signals. Afferent discharge from the spindles enhances the main spinal motor discharge to the muscle when there is a mis-match between the length set by the spindle and that achieved by the muscle. It is not known whether this afferent traffic from the spindle is accessible to higher centres as an index of muscular achievement.

Dyspnoea

This is one of the most important symptoms of respiratory disease and its mode of production is probably complex. It may be defined as an awareness of increased respiratory effort which is unpleasant and recognised as inappropriate. Dyspnoea is NOT:

1. HYPERVENTILATION

This term is reserved for breathing which is in excess of the body's needs and which therefore results in a lowering of alveolar and arterial Pco_2.

2. HYPERPNOEA

This merely indicates an increased level of ventilation, such as occurs during exercise: it is appropriate to the situation and not unpleasant.

3. TACHYPNOEA
This refers to increased rate of breathing.

Experimental work using such techniques as curarisation and local anaesthesia of the vagi and chest wall suggests that vagal input, muscular action, chest wall movement and other sensations are probably all important in the genesis of dyspnoea. There is little to suggest a single source or pathway.

Appreciation of dyspnoea involves recognition of an unsatisfactory ventilatory movement relative to the drive to breathe or an excessive drive to breathe relative to the prevailing circumstances or both. Breathing movements, drive and circumstances are in some way compared with the integrated past experience of each.

CHAPTER 3 · SURFACE TENSION AND ALVEOLAR STABILITY

Surface tension and small bubbles

Surface tension acting at the curved internal surface of a bubble tends to cause it to decrease in size. The smaller the bubble, the greater this contracting force; small bubbles tend to empty into bigger ones (Fig. 3.1, a). Very small bubbles are very unstable and tend to collapse completely. Alveoli are essentially small bubbles and surface tension would make the lungs impossibly difficult to distend if it were not for the presence of surfactant.

Surfactant

Source and nature of surfactant

Surfactant is almost certainly derived from the type II pneumocyte. It is composed of lipoprotein, largely dipalmitoyl lecithin, which is insoluble and forms a thin (probably monomolecular) layer at the air-fluid interface. The molecules probably change their orientation relative to the surface with change in the surface area of the film.

Action of surfactant

Surfactant modifies the surface tension of the alveolar fluid film. Whereas the tendency of a bubble to collapse increases as the bubble becomes smaller, surfactant has the effect of causing surface tension to fall off markedly as the size of the surface is reduced so that a small bubble remains quite stable. Small bubbles no longer empty into bigger ones but there is instead a tendency for bubbles to adjust to the same size (Fig. 3.1, c). Fluid surfaces with surfactant activity exhibit hysteresis—the surface tension—lowering effect of surfactant is improved by a transient increase in size of the surface. During quiet breathing there may be a tendency for occasional alveoli to be underventilated and gradually decrease in size. A deep breath re-expands such alveoli and restores the performance of the surfactant layer. Occasional deep breaths or sighs are a feature of normal breathing and there is some evidence that minute areas of collapse may develop if sighing is prevented. In normal individuals restriction of movement of the chest wall with strapping results in the

27

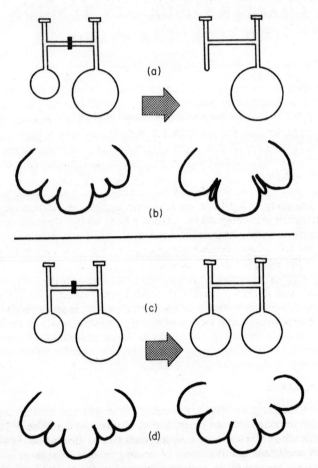

Fig. 3.1. *Surface tension and alveolar stability*

(a) *No surfactant.* Small bubbles exert greater retractive force than larger bubbles. In a closed system such as that illustrated small bubbles tend to empty into larger ones.

(b) Diagram of the equivalent situation at alveolar level. Although alveoli are not interconnected by a closed system they exert retractive forces on each other by virtue of their side-by-side and back-to-back arrangement in the lung.

(c) *Surfactant present.* Surfactant reduces surface tension as the surface area is reduced. Small bubbles then exert only a small retractive force. Larger bubbles tend to empty into them until the bubbles are of similar size.

(d) Equivalent situation at alveolar level. Small alveoli are now stable and there is a tendency for alveoli to adopt a uniform size.

development of patchy radiological collapse and an increase in intra-pulmonary shunting over the course of some hours. These effects are reversed by one or two deep breaths.

Significance of surfactant in pulmonary disease

It is difficult to measure surfactant activity quantitatively. Surfactant activity is undoubtedly defective in a number of parenchymal lung disorders but in most of these the defect is probably a consequence of lung damage rather than the cause. Defective surfactant activity plays a central role in Respiratory Distress Syndrome of the newborn and may play some part in the evolution and recovery from pulmonary oedema, lung collapse, pneumonia etc.

Patients with painful abdominal wounds, fractured ribs or thoracic cage deformity and patients on long-term artificial ventilation may have shallow tidal breathing and be prevented from taking adequate sighs. All are prone to patchy lung collapse particularly at the lung bases. It seems possible that failure to maintain surfactant activity may have some part to play in the evolution of the collapse.

Production of surfactant is impaired if pulmonary perfusion is severely reduced and this may explain the collapse associated with pulmonary embolism. A number of other factors including the presence of blood in the alveoli appear to impair surfactant activity or production.

Surfactant and the neonate

The first breath

At birth the lungs are filled with amniotic fluid. The first breaths draw the fluid-air interface into the lungs. For the infant to be able to inflate the lungs the fluid surface must have a low surface tension when the surface area is small (small bubbles must be stable). Otherwise the lungs will tend to collapse completely at every expiration. The fluid within the lungs is absorbed via the pulmonary lymphatics in the first hours of life and this is also dependent on the surface tension of the fluid being low.

Respiratory Distress Syndrome of the Newborn
(RDN, hyaline membrane disease)

PATHOGENESIS OF RDN

The syndrome is due to deficient surfactant activity usually because of prematurity. Surfactant activity is normally developed at around 32 to 35 weeks of gestation. In affected infants the alveoli have no stability and the lungs tend to collapse almost completely at the end of each expiration. Lung compliance is extremely low and the infant is unable to maintain adequate ventilation. Severe hypoxia results from underventilation, shunting of blood through airless parts of the lungs and from the re-opening of foetal right to left shunts as a consequence of hypoxic pulmonare vasoconstriction.

Autopsy specimens of lung are largely airless. Some alveolar ducts may be aerated and contain a layer of proteinaceous material—hyaline membrane—which is probably derived from plasma proteins which have leaked from damaged alveolar capillaries.

CLINICAL FEATURES

Signs of respiratory distress—tachypnoea, sternal recession, grunting, cyanosis and tachycardia—are sometimes evident from the first few minutes but may not develop until after an hour or two. The tendency is towards gradual deterioration and without treatment the mortality is very high.

MANAGEMENT

This requires specialist skills. In moderately affected babies oxygenation can be achieved by oxygen administration in an incubator. Severely affected babies require IPPV by cuffed endotracheal tube. Some improvement in results has been achieved with the use of various devices designed to maintain a slight positive pressure in the airways throughout the breathing cycle. The concentration of oxygen employed requires careful control. Sustained levels of Po_2 above 20 kPa (150 mmHg) may cause retrolental fibroplasia and pulmonary oxygen toxicity may be produced with inspired concentrations in excess of 50 per cent. Repeated measurements of arterial or capillary blood gas levels are usually necessary. Control of temperature, pH, fluid intake and feeding all require detailed attention. Progress is reflected by the concentration of oxygen required to maintain a Po_2 of about 8 kPa (60 mmHg) and by other parameters such as radiological appearances, ease of ventilation of the lungs etc.

CHAPTER 4 · THE HISTORY—
SYMPTOMS OF RESPIRATORY
DISEASE

Assessment of the patient with respiratory disease hinges on thorough, unhurried history-taking and not upon tests of pulmonary function or the chest X-ray. The aim, as in all history-taking, is to obtain a clear impression of particular symptoms and combinations of symptoms and most importantly to build up a clear picture of their progress or variation with time. The following notes are not intended to be exhaustive but they may be helpful in suggesting ways in which enquiry may be extended.

Dyspnoea (see p. 25)

CHARACTER

What words does the patient use? 'Tightness' may indicate airways obstruction or angina; 'gasping' and 'panting' suggest hyperpnoea—excessive but not necessarily laboured or obstructed breathing. The patient may liken the dyspnoea to the sensation which normally follows running. Is there accompanying noise? A wheezing sound is suggestive of airways narrowing (which may accompany disease not primarily affecting the airways such as pulmonary embolism or incipient pulmonary oedema). A frothy bubbling may accompany frank pulmonary oedema. It is often helpful when in doubt to mimic the sounds in question (wheezing can be reproduced by first breathing quietly right out almost to residual volume and then giving a further sharp forced expiration).

CIRCUMSTANCES

Is it related to time of day, exercise, meals, posture etc.? Patients with long-standing overinflation dislike bending intensely; asthma has a characteristic diurnal variation (p. 115) and so on.

HOW SEVERE IS IT?

The effect upon a patient's activities is the best guide to severity. Exercise tolerance may be crudely but usefully graded as follows:

	Grade
Short of breath at rest	4
Short of breath walking about the house and undertaking light activity such as washing	3

Grade

Has to stop even when walking at own reduced pace on
the level   2
Asks friends of own age to slow down but keeps going
at own reduced pace on level   1
Able to walk with friends at normal pace on level but
unable to keep going on hills or when hurrying   0

Useful insight may be gained into the rate and progress of disability by
noting change in a patient's *range*. When was he last shopping in a distant
centre, when last shopping locally or visiting park or pub? When was the
patient last beyond the street in which he lives, the garden gate, the front
door, one floor of the house, one room, chair or bed?

Cough and sputum

The duration and annual or daily pattern of cough and sputum production
should be clearly established. Nocturnal cough is particularly likely to be
associated with asthma or left heart failure. The approximate volume,
texture and colour of sputum should be recorded. Black particles usually
only reflect local atmospheric pollution, yellow sputum usually indicates a
high cellular content due to bacterial infection but in asthma eosinophil
clumps can produce similar appearances. Regular production of green
sputum may indicate bronchiectasis as may longstanding day-long production of large volumes of sputum. Enquiry should be made regarding
previous *haemoptysis*, its quantity and possible association with epistaxis, fever, chest pain or other respiratory symptoms.

Chest pain

The association of chest pain with respiratory movement, coughing or
turning over will suggest a pleural origin. It is sometimes helpful to mimic
the wince and grunt which an inspiration evokes in the presence of pleural
pain—this is generally recognised immediately by patients who have
experienced the symptom. Normal individuals may experience occasional
pleural pain which is transient and relieved by gradually taking a deep
breath in small steps and this phenomenon is referred to as the 'Catch
syndrome'. Sometimes localised anterior chest pain of this sort is accompanied by tenderness of one costochondral junction and this is referred to
as Tietze's syndrome or costochondritis: a benign condition. Obese
individuals are sometimes troubled by brief costal-margin pain interrupt-
ing a breath related to a rib (usually the ninth) rolling over the rib above
(clicking rib). Shoulder-tip pain suggests irritation of diaphragmatic
pleura and radiation of precordial pain to the neck and arms suggests a
myocardial origin. Precordial pain may also accompany mediastinal

enlargement, pericarditis and oesophagitis all of which may have special additional features. Pain in the epigastrium and around the costal margin is common in severe airways obstruction and may be related to peptic ulceration, oesophagitis and extreme muscular effort.

Previous respiratory illness

If a patient reports previous episodes of 'bronchitis', 'influenza', 'pneumonia' etc. it is important to obtain a clear account of the nature of the illness and not merely to accept the offered diagnosis at face value. Careful enquiry may reveal that a reported episode of 'bronchitis' had features very suggestive of asthma or that 'pneumonia' might in fact have been pulmonary embolism. The extent of previous investigations and the response to treatment may provide valuable clues. Enquiry should always be made regarding previous X-ray examinations; a surprising proportion of the adult population in the U.K. has had a chest X-ray at some time or other and, if previous films can be located, they may sometimes provide invaluable information.

Associated allergies

Allergic lung disorders, particularly asthma, are so common that enquiry should always be made about previous skin disorders (eczema, 'dermatitis'), hay fever, recurrent or persistent colds, nasal obstruction, nasal operations etc.

Family history

A similar enquiry should be made regarding allergic disorders in the family and this should be extended to include 'bronchitis' wheezing and excessive cough and breathlessness as well as tuberculosis. It is worthwhile pausing whilst the patient reviews each generation in turn; if enquiry is hurried it is very likely to be negative.

Occupational history

A clear sequential account of a patient's previous occupations including descriptions of the actual tasks and names of materials encountered may be vital (see especially Asthma, Allergic Extrinsic Alveolitis, Asbestos, Pneumoconiosis).

Smoking history

It is important to obtain a clear account of total smoking exposure and not to be misled by patients who may have recently reduced their consumption or stopped smoking.

CHAPTER 5 · EXAMINATION OF THE CHEST

Some important clues relating to the respiratory system may be evident from the moment the patient is first seen and these signs should be noted carefully lest they be overlooked during formal examination of the chest. They include the character of the breathing and its relationship to activity and speech, the shape of the shoulders (Fig. 5.1) and spine and the character of the cough. The presence of partial nasal obstruction may be apparent when the patient first speaks but is likely to be overlooked later.

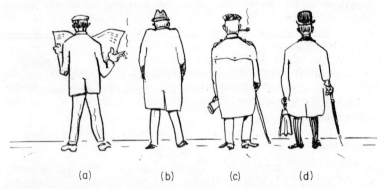

(a)   (b)   (c)   (d)

Fig. 5.1. Which man has airways obstruction? (Answer at foot of p. 37)

Inspection

Cyanosis

Cyanosis is generally apparent when about 5g/100ml of haemoglobin is present in the reduced state within the blood vessels of the skin.

PERIPHERAL CYANOSIS
Commonly due to local circulatory slowing resulting in more complete extraction of oxygen from the blood. The regions in question are commonly cool.

CENTRAL CYANOSIS
Said to exist when the bluish coloration involves areas not normally

prone to local circulatory changes. The best site to examine is the tip of the tongue. The lips may sometimes appear blue due to local pigmentation or local circulatory change but the tip of the tongue almost always has adequate blood supply. Central cyanosis indicates that there is desaturation of arterial blood. When using tissue colour to assess arterial oxygenation note should obviously be taken of the pinkest area visible. Arterial oxygenation cannot be worse than the level suggested by this area. When there is frank central cyanosis arterial Po_2 will almost always be below 6 kPa (45 mmHg) depending on haemeoglobin content and arterial pH.

Cervical neck veins

Should be inspected carefully with the patient lying between 30 and 45 degrees from the horizontal.

Clubbing

Easier to recognise than to define rigidly. There is increased curvature of the nail and the nail-bed is raised so that the normal angle between the proximal part of the nail and the skin over the dorsum of the terminal phalanx is lost (Fig. 5.2). The base of the nail may be palpable through the skin and an abnormal sponginess may be apparent when pressure is applied over it. Clubbing is associated with:
1   bronchial carcinoma
2   bronchiectasis and other forms of chronic suppurative lung disease
3   pulmonary fibrosis
4   pleural and mediastinal tumours
5   subacute bacterial endocarditis
6   cyanotic congenital heart disease
7   cirrhosis and coeliac disease.

Breathing pattern

From the beginning of the encounter with the patient there will be the opportunity to observe whether he appears to be breathless or distressed, grunting or in pain, wheezing or panting etc. and these important features should be carefully noted. If it is suspected that the respiratory rate may be increased it should be counted over a whole minute as the error inherent in counting for a shorter period such as 15 seconds is large and reduces the value of the observation, particularly if the rate is being counted serially.

Stridor

This (often sinister) sign is likely to be noticed early in the interview as the

patient draws breath whilst talking rather than during formal examination
of the chest. It can be imitated by breathing in and out with the vocal
cords held in the position of the whispered word 'air'. It indicates localised
obstruction of the larynx, trachea or large bronchi.

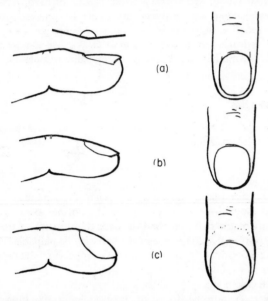

Fig. 5.2. *Clubbing.* (a) Normal, showing the 'angle'. (b) Early clubbing; the
angle is absent. (c) Advanced clubbing. The nail shows increased curvature in
all directions, the angle is absent, the base of the nail is raised up by spongy
tissue and the end of the digit is expanded.

Inspection of the chest

The chest should be carefully inspected for the presence of kyphosis,
asymmetry, overinflation etc. Use of the accessory muscles should be
noted.

Respiratory movements

Despite its semi-rigid nature the chest reflects filling of the underlying
lung in its movements remarkably well. The diseased side always moves
least. In airways obstruction of any severity it is common to note paradoxical inward movement of the costal margin during inspiration (Fig.
5.3). Where there is marked reduction of lung compliance or inspiratory
airways obstruction in-drawing of the intercostal spaces and supraclavi-
cular fossae may be observed in thin individuals.

RESTING ————————➤ INSPIRATION

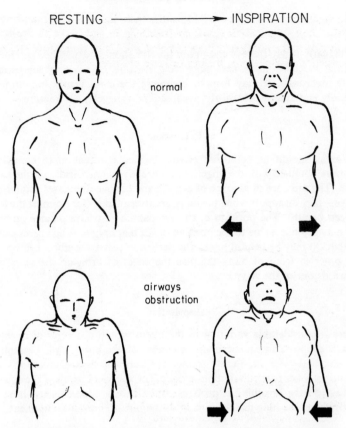

Fig. 5.3. Normally the costal margin moves *outwards* during inspiration but in the presence of substantial airways obstruction it commonly moves *inwards* and this may constitute a useful sign in a breathless patient.

Palpation

Cervical and axillary lymph nodes

These lymph nodes should always be carefully palpated.

Position of the mediastinum

This is assessed by localisation of the trachea above and the cardiac apex below.

From Fig 5.1. (b) has airways obstruction; note high position of the shoulders.

Ribs

Particularly where there is chest pain the ribs should be palpated carefully seeking localised tenderness suggesting fracture or swelling suggesting bony metastasis. It may help to compress the chest gently but firmly, laterally and antero-posteriorly; localised pain suggests rib fracture.

Percussion

All areas should be percussed paying particular attention to compare the note obtained with the finger placed exactly symmetrically on the two. sides. The presence or absence of hepatic and cardiac dullnesses should be noted—they disappear when the lungs are overinflated (for example during a deep breath). The position of the tympanitic gastric resonance on the left may provide a clue to the position of the diaphragm. When percussing the back it may be helpful to ask the patient to place one elbow on top of the other in front of him—this has the effect of bringing the scapulae forwards out of the way.

Auscultation

There is considerable variation in the intensity and character of normal breath sounds consequent upon thickness of the chest wall, breathing pattern, body size etc. Breath sounds are normally harsher anteriorly in the upper lobes particularly on the right. The source of much of the sound audible during breathing is probably turbulence produced in the larynx. Normal aerated lung filters off most of the high-frequency component.

Bronchial breathing

This can be heard over consolidated areas of lung. These areas conduct the high-frequency 'hiss' component from the larger airways quite well. Bronchial breathing is characteristically rather similar in inspiration and expiration and there is a momentary silent pause between the two. The sound can be imitated by listening with a stethoscope over the larynx whilst the subject breathes in and out with the vocal cords held in the position of a whispered 'ee'.

Added sounds (adventitiae)

Semantic difficulties arise here. The term râle is taken by some to mean any added sound and by others as synonymous with crepitation and for this reason it is perhaps best avoided.

RHONCHI

Sustained wheezing sounds of varying length and pitch. They may be heard during inspiration or expiration (more commonly the latter) and they are then produced by a flow-limiting mechanism (see p. 11). Rhonchi tend to be heard in the presence of airways obstruction but they are not inevitably present in this situation and they are generally a poor indication of the severity of the obstruction.

CREPITATIONS

A series of very brief crackling sounds which may be loud and coarse or fine and high-pitched. The sounds are probably produced by the opening of previously closed bronchioles. The timing of crepitations is of some significance.

Early inspiratory crepitations

These are associated with diffuse airways obstruction. A series of clicks are commonly heard very close together at the beginning of inspiration with relative silence afterwards. These sounds do *not* indicate pulmonary oedema, left ventricular failure etc.

Pan-inspiratory or late inspiratory crepitations

These crepitations are associated with diffuse fibrosis, pulmonary oedema (actual or incipient), bronchiectasis and partial consolidation (Fig. 5.4).

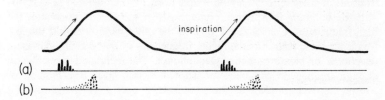

Fig. 5.4. Timing of crepitations. Diagramatic representation of (a) Early inspiratory crepitations or crackles—commonly associated with airways obstruction. (b) Pan-inspiratory or late inspiratory crepitations—commonly associated with early pulmonary oedema, lung fibrosis etc.

Probable explanation. During inspiration areas of lung open up in sequence according to their compliance (distensibility). Compliant areas open up first and then, as the retractive forces in the lung increase, increasingly stiff areas participate in receiving inspired air.

In the case of airways obstruction there may be widespread terminal airways closure during expiration particularly in relatively compliant (floppy) parts of the lung. During inspiration these areas accept air most readily and the clicks are probably produced by the opening of their airways early in inspiration.

The disorders associated with late inspiratory crepitations cause reduced lung compliance (increased stiffness) which is to some extent patchily distributed. During inspiration air passes first to the more compliant (distensible) parts—that is to the more normal parts—and only begins to enter the stiffer abnormal areas later in inspiration as lung recoil forces build up in the stretching lung.

PLEURAL RUB
Pleural rubs are commonly creaking or groaning sounds and sometimes take the form of an interrupted dry scuffing sound. They are often quite localised and indicate roughening of the normally slippery pleural surfaces.

VOCAL FREMITUS
(Included here because it concerns sound transmission.) Normal aerated lung transmits *low* frequencies well and a sonorous voice produces easily palpable fremitus (a buzzing vibration) over the chest wall. Consolidated lung transmits fremitus less well and pleural fluid very severely dampens it and may obliterate the vibrations altogether.

VOCAL RESONANCE
The character of vocal resonance—observed by auscultation over the chest during speech—provides further evidence of the lung's ability to transmit or filter different sound frequencies. Normal aerated lung transmits the booming low-pitched components of speech and attenuates the high frequencies. Consolidated lung on the other hand filters off the low frequencies and transmits the higher frequencies so that speech takes on a telephonic or bleating quality (aegophony). The facilitated transmission of high frequencies can be demonstrated by the clear transmission of whispering over consolidated lung (whispering pectriloquy). Pleural fluid reduces the intensity of all frequencies, most especially low frequencies.

THE CHARACTER OF THE COUGH
The sound produced by a cough is a most valuable (and widely ignored) physical sign. The patient should be requested to give several sharp coughs (not merely clearing the throat). A rattling sound may give clear indication of the presence of abundant bronchial secretions. A 'bovine cough' lacking the usual explosive onset may suggest vocal cord paralysis. Most importantly a muffled wheezy cough may provide a very vivid indication of the presence of otherwise quite unsuspected airways obstruction.

The sputum

The sputum should *always* be inspected. Truly clear sputum is unusual in city dwellers and if it is thin, slimy and bubbly the specimen is probably saliva. Greyish mottled fragments are usually present in true mucoid sputum. In asthma mucoid sputum may be so tenacious that it is impossible to tip it out of a container and it frequently has a glary refractile appearance. If the sputum is creamy or yellow it is referred to as purulent and this appearance commonly reflects active bronchial bacterial infection. Green- or khaki-coloured sputum indicates delay in production of sputum and suggests bronchiectasis or chronic lung abscess. Brown sputum may be produced by intra-alveolar haemorrhage or a resolving haemoptysis. Solid chunks of sputum are seen in asthma and small bronchial casts may sometimes be seen hanging like fronds below the surface if sputum is suspended in water. A transparent container is an advantage when inspecting sputum, particularly if there is a large amount of saliva and an ordinary universal container is useful in this context.

SIGNS OF LOCAL LUNG DISEASE

Certain distinctive combinations of physical signs have for generations been recognised as allowing some crude assessment of the type of gross pathological change within the chest. The correlation between the signs and the underlying changes is much looser than is the case in cardiological examination and it is as well to be aware of the limitations of physical examination. In developed countries it is realistic to regard the chest X-ray as a normal extension of physical examination. In the case of localised lung disease the appearances of the chest X-ray frequently modify the interpretation of the physical signs.

Signs of consolidation (airless but not collapsed lung)

Movement of the affected side may be less.
Percussion note is dull—not usually profoundly so.
Vocal fremitus may be somewhat reduced.
Bronchial breathing may be heard.
Crepitations may be heard (pan-inspiratory or late inspiratory).
Vocal resonance may have a bleating quality (aegophony).
Whispering pectriloquy may be heard.

SUMMARY
Moderate dullness, often crepitations and characteristically well-conducted high-pitched sound.

Signs of collapse

Reduction in lung volume may be apparent from movement of the *trachea* towards the collapsed side. The chest wall may appear flattened on the affected side. The apex may be displaced towards the collapse. Movement of the affected side may be reduced. The gastric resonance may be exceptionally high in left-sided collapse.

Breath sounds are usually diminished over the collapsed lobe. In addition to these signs there may be signs of consolidation as outlined above— collapse and consolidation commonly occur together.

Note. These signs may be present in massive collapse but sometimes negligible signs accompany collapse particularly of a lower lobe.

SUMMARY
Perhaps evidence of localised loss of lung volume with reduction in movement, breath sounds and moderate dullness on percussion.

Signs of pleural effusion

Trachea and apex may be displaced away from the effusion if it is massive.

Movement of the affected side may be reduced.

Dullness on percussion. This is the most important sign of pleural fluid and is maximal at the base and in the axilla. At least 500 ml of fluid seem to be necessary before dullness becomes detectable.

Vocal fremitus is reduced or absent over pleural fluid.

Breath sounds are reduced or absent. Towards the upper part of an effusion there may be signs of consolidation.

SUMMARY
Striking dullness on percussion with reduction of breath sounds and vocal fremitus.

Signs of pneumothorax

WITHOUT TENSION
In a small pneumothorax there may be *no* signs at all.

Percussion is usually unremarkable ('hyperresonance' is usually unconvincing).

Breath sounds are absent or much reduced and this may be the only sign. A clicking sound in time with the heart is sometimes heard in small left-sided pneumothoraces due to intermittent contact of the two pleural surfaces over the heart. Other signs are generally lacking.

TENSION PNEUMOTHORAX

Trachea and apex are displaced away from the affected side (important).

Movement of the side may be reduced and the chest may appear fuller on that side.

Percussion may yield a hyperresonant note.

Breath sounds are absent over the pneumothorax.

Vocal resonance and fremitus are somewhat reduced. Tachypnoea and respiratory distress are usual and there may be hypotension, sweating and congestion of neck veins.

SUMMARY

Absent or reduced breath sounds without dullness or signs of consolidation. In tension pneumothorax: displacement of the mediastinum, reduced movement, overdistension and signs of circulatory embarrassment.

Signs of pleural thickening

This is difficult to diagnose with certainty from signs alone.

Movement of the side may be reduced if thickening is extensive.

Dullness on percussion is usual but may not be striking.

Breath sounds are reduced.

Vocal resonance and fremitus are impaired.

Other signs: a pleural rub may be audible but other signs are generally lacking.

SUMMARY

Signs suggestive of a small pleural effusion with sometimes reduced movement of the side in question.

Signs of local pulmonary fibrosis

This is difficult to distinguish from collapse. Upper lobe fibrosis (usually related to old tuberculosis) may produce deviation of the trachea towards the affected side with flattening and reduced movement of the upper chest. Slight dullness, bronchial breathing and crepitations may be evident over the upper lobe.

SIGNS OF DIFFUSE LUNG DISEASE

Diffuse pulmonary fibrosis—p. 141.

Pulmonary oedema—p. 202.

Bronchiectasis—p. 100.

Signs of diffuse airways obstruction

Recognition depends upon the history and physical findings as the chest X-ray is generally unhelpful. The diagnosis does **not** hinge upon the finding of rhonchi on auscultation.

The character of the cough is wheezy or muffled—a convenient and very valuable sign.

Signs of overinflation. These can be mimicked by taking in a full breath when it will be found that:

1   The shoulders are high (Fig. 5.1).
2   The antero-posterior diameter of the chest is increased.
3   Accessory muscles of respiration are in operation.
4   Further expansion is limited and accompanied by *inward* movement of the costal margin (Fig. 5.3) and sometimes by descent of the larynx.
5   Percussion reveals absent hepatic and cardiac dullness.

Breathing pattern. In severe airways obstruction the patient appears to snatch at inspiration and to have a (relatively) prolonged expiration. In less severe obstruction prolonged expiration is not very obvious.

Rhonchi. These may be of high or low pitch and tend to be more marked towards the end of expiration.

Note. Very severe airways obstruction can exist without rhonchi. The loudness of ronchi is related to breathing pattern and is a very poor indicator of severity of obstruction. Prominent inspiratory rhonchi are suggestive of asthma.

Crepitations. Early inspiratory crepitations and clicks may be heard (p. 39, Fig. 5.4).

Prolonged forced expiratory time. A maximum forced expiration from a position of full inspiration can normally be completed within about 5 seconds. Prolongation beyond this time generally indicates airways obstruction. The end of expiration can be determined by auscultation over the trachea.

CHAPTER 6 · PULMONARY FUNCTION TESTS

Despite the bewildering profusion of sophisticated investigations now employed in testing pulmonary function it (happily) remains possible to obtain most of the information relevant to clinical practice with the aid of a few fairly simple tests. In this section the emphasis will be on simplicity and practicality.

SIMPLE TESTS OF VENTILATORY FUNCTION

Ventilation refers to the process of moving air into and out of the lungs.

Normal values

Ventilatory performance varies widely with body size, age and sex (Fig. 6.1). Tables and nomograms are available which take these variables into account and display 'predicted normal values' for individuals of particular age and height. These 'predicted' values are the *mean* values derived from study of a normal population and it should be understood that there is considerable variation about this mean (Fig. 6.2). For example the standard deviation of the mean predicted value for vital capacity is about 500 ml. In effect this means that if a medium-sized adult has a vital capacity which is one litre below the predicted normal value the low result *may* be the result of respiratory disease but on the other hand the value is only just 2 standard deviations from the mean and perhaps 5 per cent of normal individuals of the same age and size will be found to have a lower vital capacity than this. The practice of expressing results as a 'percentage of predicted normal' is thus potentially misleading: the finding of a vital capacity of 75 per cent of the predicted value does not indicate a 25 per cent disability and is still compatible with normality.

Vital capacity

The vital capacity is the volume of air expelled by a maximal expiration from a position of full inspiration and this can be measured with any spirometer (Fig. 6.3).

Vital capacity is reduced in the following circumstances:

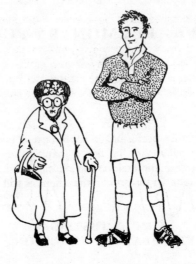

FEV$_1$	1·12	4·32	(litres)
FVC	1·60	5·80	(litres)

Fig. 6.1. Normal values!

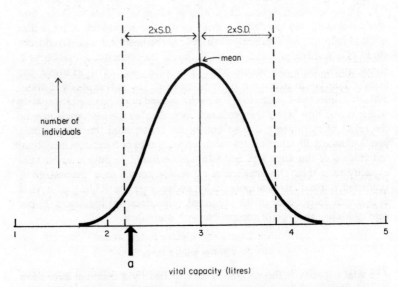

Fig. 6.2. Distribution of Vital Capacity in normal individuals of one particular age height and sex (see text).

1 Reduced lung compliance (lung fibrosis, infiltration, loss of lung volume, pulmonary oedema etc.).

2 Deformity of the chest (kyphoscoliosis, ankylosing spondylitis etc.).

3 Muscular weakness (myopathy, myasthenia gravis etc.).

4 Airways obstruction. (Although the main defect is a limitation in rate of air-flow, reduction in vital capacity is almost inevitable.)

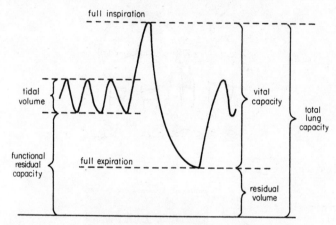

Fig. 6.3. The more commonly used subdivisions of total lung capacity.

Peak Expiratory Flow Rate (PEFR)

This is measured with a peak flow meter or a peak flow gauge (Fig. 6.4). It is the maximum *rate* of air-flow which can be achieved during a sudden forced expiration from a position of full inspiration. The best of three attempts is usually accepted as the PEFR. The value achieved is a little dependent on effort but is mainly determined by the calibre of the airways. The importance of lung volume in determining maximal expiratory air-flow has already been mentioned (p. 8) and it follows from this that it is essential that the forced expiration should be performed from the full inspiratory position. The results must be related to body size. PEFR is particularly impaired in the presence of diffuse airways obstruction but it is also somewhat impaired in conditions which reduce lung volume.

The Forced Expiratory Volume in one second (FEV$_1$) and the Forced Vital Capacity (FVC)

The FEV$_1$ is the volume of air expelled in the first second of a maximal forced expiration from a position of full inspiration. The forced vital capacity is obtained by continuing the forced expiration until no further air can be expelled.

The FEV_1 is reduced in any condition which reduces vital capacity but it is particularly reduced when there is diffuse airways obstruction. The relationship between FEV_1 and FVC is clinically very useful as it is to a large extent independent of body size and age.

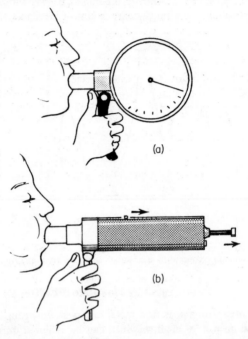

Fig. 6.4. *Measurement of Peak Expiratory Flow Rate (PEFR).* (a) Wright Peak Flow Meter; (b) Peak Flow Gauge. Both manufactured by Air Med, Clement Clarke International.

The subject takes a *full inspiration*, applies the lips to the mouthpiece and delivers a *sudden* maximal expiratory blast. In (a) a spring-loaded vane is pushed by the expired air uncovering a slot through which air escapes. A ratchet retains the vane at its furthest excursion and PEFR is read from the dial which is calibrated in litres per minute. In (b) the vane is replaced by a piston which uncovers a slot at the top of the cylinder. A ratchet retains the piston at its point of maximum excursion and PEFR is read from a scale on the top of the cylinder. Good agreement is obtained between results obtained with the two instruments.

In a forced expiration about 75 per cent of the air is expelled in the first second ($FEV_1/FVC = 0.75$, this is sometimes referred to as the forced expiratory ratio). In the presence of diffuse airways obstruction a smaller proportion of the air is expelled in the first second (the forced expiratory ratio is reduced).

'Restrictive' and 'obstructive' patterns of ventilatory impairment

When lung volume is restricted by pulmonary fibrosis or infiltration or by rigidity of the chest wall the VC is reduced and the FEV_1 is also reduced in proportion and the forced expiratory ratio is normal or even higher than normal. This pattern of ventilatory impairment is described as a restrictive defect.

In the presence of airways obstruction VC and FEV_1 are again reduced but the FEV_1 is proportionately greater affected than the VC. The forced expiratory ratio is reduced and this pattern is referred to as an obstructive defect.

The forced expiratory spirogram

Any spirometer equipped with a fast-moving recording chart may be used to record the forced expiratory spirogram from which the FEV_1 and FVC may be read. It is important that a true maximum forced expiration is achieved. This can be checked by observing the striking reproducibility of the true forced expiratory spirogram. The FEV_1 and FVC are generally taken as the best of 3 closely reproducible attempts. Comparison of successive attempts and other useful features of the spirogram can be observed most readily with spirometers which are equipped to start the

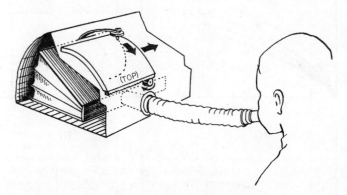

Fig. 6.5. *Schematic view of Vitalograph dry spirometer*
The main components are a bellows and a moving record chart. An arm attached to the bellows carries a writing point which moves forwards across the chart as air enters the bellows. As soon as the bellows moves a microswitch is triggered and a motor causes the record chart to move steadily from left to right. The combination of lateral movement of the chart and forward movement of the writing point causes an oblique line to be inscribed upon the chart (see Fig. 6.6).

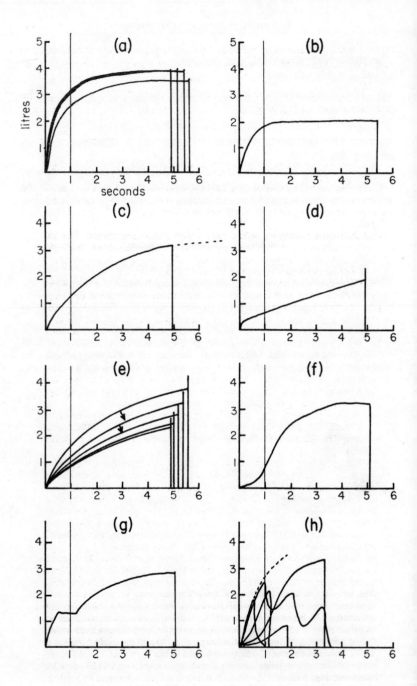

expired tracing at the same point at each attempt. A widely available self-triggering bellows-type spirometer (Vitalograph) possesses this important facility as well as a number of other features of practical importance (Fig. 6.5). Some commonly encountered patterns of forced expiratory spirogram are shown in Fig. 6.6.

Fig. 6.6. *Forced expiratory spirogram tracings obtained with a Vitalograph spirometer.*

(a) *Normal.* Four expirations have been made. Three of these were true maximal forced expirations as indicated by their *reproducibility*. The FEV_1 is 3·2 litres and the VC is 3·8 litres. The forced expiratory ratio (FEV_1/VC) is 84 per cent.

(b) *Restrictive ventilatory defect.* Patient with pulmonary fibrosis. The VC in this case was 2 litres less than the predicted value for the subject. The FEV_1 is also reduced below the predicted value but it represents a large part of the VC. Forced expiratory ratio is greater than 90 per cent.

(c) *Obstructive ventilatory defect.* The FEV_1 is much reduced. The rate of air-flow is severely reduced as indicated by the reduced slope of the curve. Note that the forced expiratory time is increased—the patient is still blowing out at 5 seconds. The vital capacity has not been adequately recorded in this case because the patient did not continue the expiration after the chart stopped moving; he could have expired further (this is a common technical error).

(d) *Severe airways obstruction.* The FEV_1 is about 0·5 litres. VC is also reduced but not so strikingly as FEV_1. Forced expiratory ratio 23 per cent. Very low expiratory flow rate. This pattern of a very brief initial rapid phase followed by a straight line indicating little change in maximal flow rate with change in lung volume is sometimes associated with severe emphysema.

(e) *Airways obstruction and bronchial hyperreactivity.* Five expirations have been made. FEV_1 and VC become lower with each expiration. Patient with asthma. This feature suggests poor control of asthma and liability to severe attacks.

(f) *A non-maximal expiration.* Compare with (a). In a true forced expiration the steepest part of the curve always occurs at the beginning of expiration which is not the case in (f). A falsely low FEV_1 and forced expiratory ratio are obtained. Usually the patient has not understood what is required or is unable to co-ordinate his actions. Occasional patients wish to appear worse than they really are. This pattern is unlikely to be mistaken for a true forced expiration because of its shape and because it cannot be reproduced repeatedly.

(g) *Escape of air* from either the nose or lips during expiration.

(h) *Inability to perform the manœuvre.* Five attempts have been made. In some the patient has breathed in and out. Other attempts are either not maximal forced expirations or are unfinished. Bizarre patterns such as this are often seen in patients with psychogenic breathlessness and in the elderly and demented. Even with poor co-operation it is often possible to obtain useful information. In the example shown (h) significant airways obstruction can be excluded because of the steep slope of at least two of the expirations which follow an identical course and show appropriate curvature (dotted line) and the VC can be estimated as not less than 3·2 litres.

Note: VC in this section is actually *forced* vital capacity (or FVC) Especially in airways obstruction VC performed slowly is rather larger than forced VC.

ALVEOLAR VENTILATION

The only satisfactory means of assessing the adequacy of ventilation is measurement of alveolar or arterial P_{CO_2} (see p. 16).

1. Measurement of P_{CO_2} by rebreathing technique

Changes in arterial P_{CO_2} are mirrored by changes in mixed venous P_{CO_2} (provided CO_2 production and cardiac output are not grossly disturbed). The rebreathing technique first described by Campbell and Howell permits mixed venous P_{CO_2} to be measured quickly and conveniently at the bedside or in the consulting room by non-invasive means (Fig. 6.7).

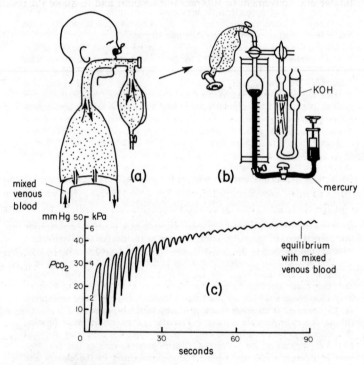

Fig. 6.7. Rebreathe P_{CO_2}.

Procedure (abbreviated version of the method)

1   A rubber bag is filled with about 2 litres of oxygen.
2   The patient breathes quietly in and out of the bag for 90 seconds.

3   The CO_2 concentration of the mixture in the bag is measured using a modified Haldane apparatus.

During the period of rebreathing the concentration of CO_2 in the bag rises sharply to start with but only very slowly towards the end of 90 seconds (Fig. 6.7). By this time there is equilibrium (with respect to CO_2) between the blood in the pulmonary capillaries (mixed venous blood) and the air going back and forth between bag and lungs. Mixed venous PCO_2 is then the same as the PCO_2 of the contents of the bag. The latter is obtained by multiplying the percentage concentration of CO_2 in the bag by the available barometric pressure (barometric pressure less water vapour pressure at $37\,°C$).

The mixed venous PCO_2 measured by this means is about 1·2 kPa (9 mmHg) higher than the arterial PCO_2. For most clinical purposes it is justifiable and convenient to subtract this amount and to quote the result as an 'arterial' PCO_2 (rebreathe method).

Arterial PCO_2 is normally between 4·8 and 6·1 kPa (36 and 46 mmHg).

2. The Astrup technique

This technique involves the measurement of arterial (or capillary) blood pH with a microelectrode. PCO_2 and bicarbonate concentration are calculated after observing the change in pH of the sample when it is exposed to gases of differing PCO_2.

Background

If a solution of bicarbonate is brought into equilibrium with several gas mixtures in turn, each with a different PCO_2, and if hydrogen ion concentration ([H^+]) is measured after each equilibration it will be found that there is a direct relationship between PCO_2 and [H^+] (Fig. 6.8). This relationship between PCO_2 and [H^+] is the basis of the Astrup method.

If some bicarbonate is added to the solution and the same procedure repeated it will again be found that there is a direct relationship between PCO_2 and [H^+] but at each level of PCO_2 the [H^+] will be lower than previously (b in Fig. 6.8).

[H^+] is generally expressed as pH which is the negative logarithm of [H^+] but this does not prevent a convenient linear plot of pH against PCO_2 if the latter is given a logarithmic scale (Fig. 6.9). For any particular bicarbonate solution a line may be plotted which describes the relationship between pH and PCO_2 in that solution.

Procedure

1   An arterial or capillary blood sample is taken (see p. 59).
2   pH of the sample is measured with minimum delay.

3   Some of the remaining blood is equilibrated in a tonometer with a gas mixture of known low P_{CO_2} and the pH then measured.

4   Some more of the remaining blood is equilibrated with a gas mixture of a known higher P_{CO_2} and the pH measured.

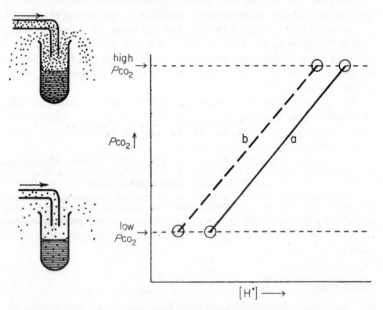

Fig. 6.8. *Astrup 1.* Relationship between P_{CO_2} and hydrogen ion concentration in a bicarbonate solution. A solution of bicarbonate is equilibrated with two gases of known P_{CO_2}. H^+ is measured. (a) shows the relationship between P_{CO_2} and H^+ for that solution (the buffer line). (b) shows the relationship for a solution with a higher bicarbonate concentration.

The Plot

The results are plotted on specially prepared paper which has axes representing pH and $\log P_{CO_2}$ as described. First the points representing the pH and P_{CO_2} of the two equilibrated samples are identified and a line is drawn through these points. Next the pH of the original sample is referred to and the line is marked at the point that it intersects with this pH. The P_{CO_2} of the original sample can now be found by referring to the vertical P_{CO_2} axis.

The position of the line has already been noted to be dependent upon the bicarbonate content of the solution. The bicarbonate content can be read directly from a horizontal nomogram.

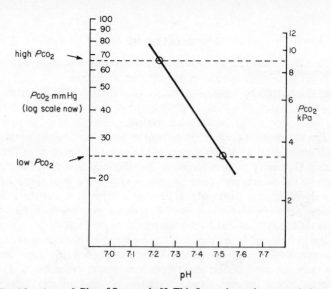

Fig. 6.9a. *Astrup 2.* Plot of P_{CO_2} and pH. This figure shows the same relationship as in Fig. 6.9a. The [H+] scale has been converted into the more widely used pH. pH is the negative logarithm of [H+]. High [H+] is now on the left and low [H+] on the right and the buffer line now slopes the other way. Because pH is a logarithmic term, P_{CO_2} has been given a logarithmic scale so that the straightline relationship between the two is retained.

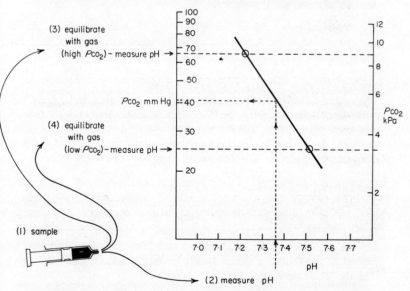

Fig. 6.9b. *Astrup 3. Procedure.* (1) An arterial or capillary sample is taken. (2) The pH of the sample is measured. (3) Part of the sample is equilibrated with a gas of known high P_{CO_2} and the pH measured. (4) Part is equilibrated with a gas of known low P_{CO_2} and the pH measured. The relationship between P_{CO_2} and pH in the sample (buffer line) is plotted from 3 and 4. Interpolation of the pH value obtained (2) allows the P_{CO_2} of the original sample to be estimated (dotted line).

Information obtained

Arterial or capillary   pH
                           P_{CO_2}
                           Bicarbonate content.

The bicarbonate content can be read as actual bicarbonate or standard bicarbonate. The actual bicarbonate concentration varies with P_{CO_2} because CO_2 reacts to produce some bicarbonate. Standard bicarbonate refers to the bicarbonate concentration which would exist if the solution were equilibrated to a P_{CO_2} of 5·33 kPa (40 mmHg). It is probably easier to become familiar with the standard bicarbonate; no allowances have to be made for the P_{CO_2} at which the measurements were made.

Buffer base and base excess can also be obtained by reference to curved nomograms (Siggaard-Andersen). These expressions recognise the fact that there are other buffers apart from bicarbonate in the blood. There is little to choose between these parameters of the buffering capacity of blood—standard bicarbonate, buffer base and base excess—it is a matter of individual preference which is employed. They all behave in a similar fashion in disturbances of acid/base homeostasis.

Analysis of acid/base disturbances

The graphical treatment of the relationship between pH, P_{CO_2} and bicarbonate used in the Astrup technique provides a convenient basis for displaying and interpreting acid/base disturbances.

RESPIRATORY ACIDOSIS AND ALKALOSIS
Changes in alveolar ventilation alter the P_{CO_2} and the arterial point will move up or down along the line (Fig. 6.10). The changes in pH are entirely due to changes in P_{CO_2} and the bicarbonate-linked indices all remain unchanged. A rise in P_{CO_2} produces a 'respiratory' acidosis and a fall in P_{CO_2} due to hyperventilation causes a 'respiratory' alkalosis.

METABOLIC ACIDOSIS AND ALKALOSIS
A change in the bicarbonate concentration of the blood through metabolic causes (e.g. diabetic ketoacidosis, renal failure etc.) results in a lateral shift of the line. A fall in plasma bicarbonate level results in movement of the line to the left. If the P_{CO_2} remains unaltered this disturbance may be termed a 'metabolic' acidosis. Excess of bicarbonate would result in a 'metabolic' alkalosis (Fig. 6.11).

COMPENSATORY CHANGES
A primary disturbance of P_{CO_2} may be compensated for by change in bicarbonate concentration and vice versa. For example in a primary

metabolic acidosis ventilation is stimulated and the P_{CO_2} falls tending to minimise the disturbance of pH. This respiratory compensation although incomplete is very prompt.

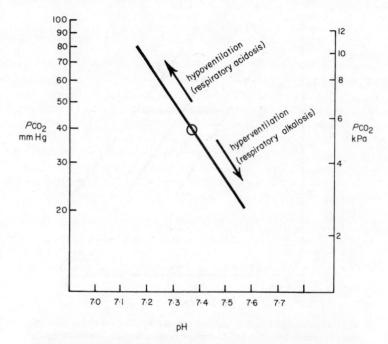

Fig. 6.10. *Astrup 4. 'Respiratory' acidosis and alkalosis.* If the bicarbonate concentration remains unaltered then changes in pH of the blood must be due to changes in P_{CO_2}. P_{CO_2} is determined by alveolar ventilation. Hyperventilation causes fall in P_{CO_2} and a rise in pH and movement of the arterial point downwards along the buffer line as shown above. Hypoventilation causes increase in P_{CO_2} and an upward movement of the arterial point.

In a primary respiratory acidosis there is increased renal reabsorption of bicarbonate which tends to minimise the disturbance of pH. Renal compensation is sluggish and takes days to develop.

MIXED DISTURBANCES

Quite commonly respiratory and metabolic disturbances occur together from separate causes. They may tend to minimise disturbance of pH in the manner of the compensatory changes described above or they may cause additive disturbance of pH. Perhaps the commonest example of an additive disturbance is the combination of respiratory acidosis due to acute

respiratory failure with metabolic acidosis due to circulatory failure
(which causes hypoxic lactic acidosis).

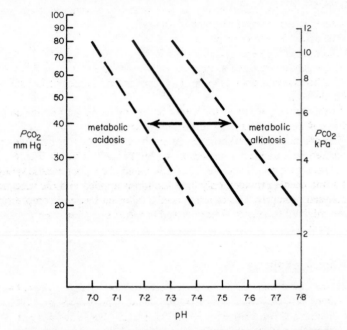

Fig. 6.11. *Astrup 5. 'Metabolic' acidosis and alkalosis.* The position of the buffer
line has already been noted to be dependent upon the bicarbonate concentration of the solution. Changes in the level of plasma bicarbonate are the result
of non-respiratory metabolic changes. pH change which is largely the result
of altered bicarbonate buffering is loosely referred to as 'metabolic'. The buffer
line moves to the left with fall in bicarbonate (metabolic acidosis) and to the
right with increase in bicarbonate (metabolic alkalosis). In the Siggaard-
Andersen plot of P_{CO_2} and pH various indices which reflect bicarbonate
content and buffering capacity of the blood can be read directly from the
intersection of the line with special nomograms.

3. The CO_2 electrode (Severinghaus type)

This provides a convenient method for measuring the P_{CO_2} of blood
samples directly. In essence it comprises a pH electrode with a thin film of
bicarbonate kept in position over its tip by a polypropylene membrane and
fitted into a small sample chamber. When blood comes into contact with
the membrane CO_2 diffuses rapidly across into the bicarbonate solution
and the pH in the solution stabilises at a value related to the sample P_{CO_2}.
The meter is calibrated to read P_{CO_2} directly and the electrode is calibrated using gases or solutions of known P_{CO_2}.

A note on arterial blood sampling

Sampling from the radial artery at the wrist has advantages over other sites such as the femoral or brachial arteries:

1 The artery is readily palpable.
2 There is no big vein accompanying it.
3 It is easily compressed against the radius after puncture.
4 If a haematoma does develop it is soon detected and not hidden beneath clothes.
5 In the unlikely event of the artery becoming damaged there is an excellent collateral circulation via the palmar arch.

There is no need to transfix the artery by a vertical stab; it may easily be entered by an angled approach along the line of the vessel (Fig. 6.12). For clinical purposes it is perfectly acceptable to use a small plastic syringe and a fine needle provided only light suction is applied and the specimen is analysed promptly. Use of a fine needle followed by good compression causes minimal trauma to the artery and repeated sampling from the same site is possible.

Capillary blood sampling

Capillary blood sampled from a warmed ear-lobe or finger yields blood gas values very close to those of arterial blood. The samples are collected into heparinised capillary tubes which are sealed. The method is not suitable when the peripheral circulation is impaired.

ARTERIAL OXYGENATION

Arterial oxygenation can be assessed by measurement of either oxygen tension or saturation.

Oxygen tension (P_{O_2})

This is measured using a Clark-type platinum polarigraphic electrode which comprises a platinum cathode and a silver anode in a tiny electrolytic cell biased by a small voltage and separated from the blood sample by a thin membrane. The current output of the cell is proportional to the availability of oxygen molecules at the platinum surface and hence to P_{O_2}.

Oxygen saturation

Saturation is generally measured using spectrophotometric methods based on the different absorption of light of particular wave lengths by reduced and oxygenated haemoglobin—a difference which is apparent from the difference in colour. In some instruments the intensity of the light transmitted through the specimen is measured and in others the reflected light is measured. The Kipp haemoreflectometer is a robust and practical example of the latter type.

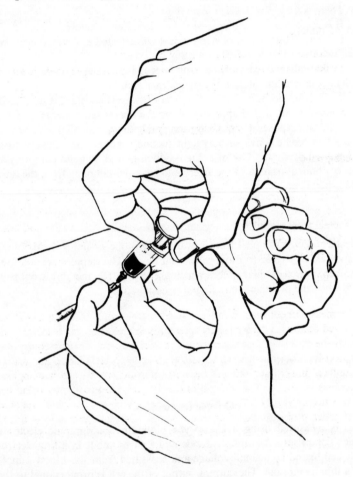

Fig. 6.12. Sampling arterial blood from radial artery.

Saturation or tension?

There is little to choose between the two forms of oxygen measurement up to a Po_2 of about 9·3 kPa (70 mmHg) and one may be obtained from the other if the pH of the blood is known. Oxygen tension is more widely used, perhaps because it is also useful in the higher range above a Po_2 of 70 mmHg where saturation hardly changes at all.

SI Units—pressure

The unit of pressure employed is the kilopascal (kPa) which is equivalent to 7·5 mmHg.

To convert kPa to mmHg multiply by 7·5
To convert mmHg to kPa multiply by 0·13 (add a third and divide by 10)

A nomogram relating kPa and mmHg appears as an appendix (p. 232).

TRANSFER FACTOR

Background

The important influence of ventilation/perfusion relationships upon gas exchange has already been noted. At one time the ability of gases to diffuse across the alveolar-capillary membrane was thought to be the principal factor limiting gas exchange in disease. This led to the concept of 'diffusing capacity'—a measurement of the rate at which gas passes from the alveoli to the bloodstream.

Diffusing capacity = quantity of gas transported across in each minute for every unit of pressure gradient.

The measurement was found to be clinically useful. Later when it was realised that many factors apart from diffusion affected gas transfer in the lungs the expression was renamed 'Transfer Factor'. Oxygen transport is obviously of most interest to clinicians but special difficulties are encountered in studying this gas because transport stops when haemoglobin becomes saturated. The difficulties can be partly overcome by using very low concentrations of oxygen which do not permit saturation of the blood but other problems are then encountered. Carbon monoxide is usually employed in the measurement of transfer factor. Very low concentrations are used so that the blood remains avid for the gas during its passage through the pulmonary capillary.

Outline of measurement

Two pieces of information are required:
1 The quantity of CO transferred per minute.
2 The pressure gradient across the alveolar membrane (this is in effect the alveolar partial pressure of CO as blood CO tension can be ignored).

Steady-state method

The patient breathes air containing a known low concentration of CO from a Douglas bag and expired air is collected in another Douglas bag over a timed period of some minutes. The rate of CO transfer (1) can be calculated from the difference between inspired and expired concentrations. The alveolar CO level (2) is more difficult to establish because it varies during each breath as CO is lost into the blood. A mean alveolar level can be calculated by estimating deadspace ventilation for CO_2 and assuming that this same volume was filled with unchanged inspired CO mixture. The short-fall in expired CO must then be entirely due to a lower concentration in the alveolar fraction which can be calculated.

Single-breath method

This is more widely used. The patient takes a measured breath containing small amounts of both helium and CO, holds the breath for 10 seconds and then breathes out. A sample of expired air is obtained (after the initial deadspace air has escaped) and the concentration of CO is measured.

The expired concentration of helium is lower than the inspired because it has been diluted by mixture with air already in the lungs at the beginning of the breath (but, being insoluble, no actual absorption has occurred). The volume of air in the lungs during the breath-hold can be calculated. The expired concentration of CO is also lower than the inspired level but the fall is proportionately greater than in the case of helium because some CO has been absorbed into the bloodstream.

The calculation of the rate of CO transfer (1) and alveolar CO tension (2) is based on the assumption that the CO is instantly diluted in the same proportion as He at the beginning of the breath-hold and that the alveolar CO concentration then falls exponentially towards the expired level (Fig. 6.13). Integration yields an expression of the relationship between rate of fall of concentration of CO and alveolar concentration of CO. When account is taken of the volume of air involved the rate of CO transfer in ml per minute per mmHg partial pressure of CO can readily be calculated.

Transfer factor is normally of the order of 20 ml/min/mmHg and is related to age, sex and body size. Transfer factor in SI units is expressed as mmol min^{-1} kPa^{-1} and is normally of the order of 6·7 mmol min^{-1} kPa^{-1}. To convert from SI units to 'old' units multiply by 3.

The significance of transfer factor

Transfer factor is influenced by many considerations which include:
1   Ventilation/perfusion imbalance—in disease much of the inspired gas may not reach perfused alveoli.

2 The thickness of the alveolar-capillary membrane.
3 The area of the membrane.
4 The pulmonary capillary blood volume.
5 The haemoglobin concentration.
6 The rate of reaction of CO with haemoglobin.

Impairment of transfer factor does not necessarily mean impairment of diffusion. Despite the number of factors which perturb it, transfer factor remains an extremely useful measurement (the same could be said of the E.S.R.).

In the presence of normal ventilatory function the finding of a significantly reduced transfer factor is a strong indication of the presence of a parenchymal lung disorder involving the alveoli or their blood supply.

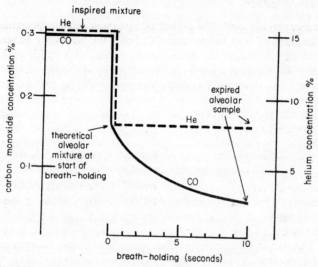

Fig. 6.13. Measurement of Transfer Factor by the single-breath method. Schematic representation of the helium and carbon monoxide concentrations in the inspired mixture and in alveolar air during breath-holding.

In the presence of a restrictive ventilatory defect an impairment of transfer factor suggests fibrosis, oedema or infiltration if the reduction is more severe than would be expected from simple reduction in lung volume (e.g. in collapse, after pneumonectomy etc.). In diffuse parenchymal disease measurement of transfer factor may provide a useful index of severity and progress.

The significance of impairment of transfer factor in the presence of an obstructive ventilatory defect is more difficult to assess and depends to some extent on the relative severity of the two defects and upon clinical circumstances. Persistent impairment of transfer factor may provide support for a diagnosis of emphysema.

EXERCISE TESTS

Exercise tests may provide valuable insight into the performance of the cardio-respiratory apparatus as a whole. Often very useful information may be obtained by merely walking with a patient on the level or up stairs. More precise information is obtained if pulse, minute ventilation and oxygen uptake are measured during graded exercise using an ergometer. Measurement of maximum exercise tolerance is useful but not without hazard in the elderly and those with cardiac disease. It is sometimes helpful to measure arterial blood gas tensions or steady-state transfer factor during exercise particularly when the cause of dyspnoea is obscure.

SUMMARY OF THE BASIC TESTS OF PULMONARY FUNCTION

PEFR	Wright Peak Flow Meter	Allows detection of major airways obstruction.
FVC FEV$_1$	Spirometer, e.g. Vitalograph	Permits recognition of defects of ventilation and provides information about their nature e.g. obstructive or restrictive.
P_{CO_2}	Rebreathing method, Astrup or CO_2 electrode	Allows assessment of alveolar ventilation. Astrup method gives information relating to acid/base status.
Transfer factor	Steady-state or single-breath methods	Provides useful non-specific information relating to gas-transfer function of the lungs which may not be readily gained by other means.
Exercise testing		Assessment of global cardio-pulmonary performance.

CHAPTER 7 · ELEMENTS OF
RADIOLOGY OF THE CHEST

The interpretation of physical signs particularly of local disease is a valuable skill but far from infallible and the ready availability of chest radiography in developed countries makes it important that the clinician
should be familiar with the elements of interpreting chest radiographs
almost as an extension of physical examination.

The normal chest X-ray

Some of the more useful landmarks of the normal chest X-ray are
indicated in Fig. 7.1. It is desirable that the film should be examined
systematically to avoid missing useful information. The centring and pene-
tration of the film should be quickly noted as these factors have considerable influence on the shape of the heart and mediastinum and upon the
character of the vascular markings in the lung fields. The shape and bony
structures of the chest wall should be surveyed and the position of the
diaphragms and trachea noted. The heart's shape and size and the appearance of the mediastinum and hilar shadows are examined. On the right side
the horizontal fissure is a particularly useful landmark and should be
carefully identified. The size, shape and disposition of the vascular shadows
are next noted and the pattern of the lung markings in different zones
carefully compared. Whenever a localised abnormality of any sort is
evident or suspected a lateral film becomes essential for accurate localisation. The main features of the lateral film are indicated in Fig. 7.2.

Collapse

Collapse of a lobe is usually evident from shift of landmarks (fissures,
mediastinum, blood vessels) and the collapsed lobe itself may cast a
characteristic shadow (Fig. 7.3.)

CONSOLIDATION
Consolidated areas of lung appear as uniform areas of opacification
which conform to the outline of a lobe or segment; there is often a variable
amount of collapse present.

Pleural effusion

Small pleural effusions (of 300–500 ml) cause no more than blunting of a

costophrenic angle; larger effusions cast a characteristic shadow with a
curved upper edge rising into the axilla (even though the upper level in

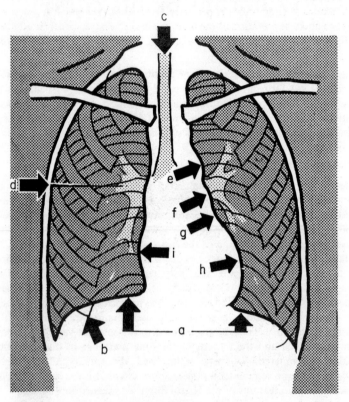

Fig. 7.1. *Diagram of chest X-ray (PA view)*
The right hemidiaphragm is 1–3 cm higher than the left (a) and on full inspiration it is intersected by the shadow of the anterior part of the sixth rib (b).
The trachea (c) is vertical and central or very slightly to the right. The horizontal fissure (d) is found in the position shown or slightly lower and should be
truly horizontal. It is a very valuable marker of change in volume of any part
of the right lung. The left border of the cardiac shadow comprises: (e) aorta;
(f) pulmonary artery; (g) concavity overlying the left atrial appendage; (h)
left ventricle. The right border of the cardiac shadow normally overlies the
right atrium (i) and above that the superior vena cava.

fact runs horizontally round the chest wall). Very large effusions cause
uniform opacification of one side of the chest and there may be shift of
the mediastinum towards the opposite side.

Fibrosis

Localised fibrosis causes streaky shadows with evidence of traction upon neighbouring structures. Upper lobe fibrosis causes traction upon the trachea and also elevation of the hilar vascular shadows. Generalised inter-stitial fibrosis produces a hazy shadowing, sometimes with a fine reticular

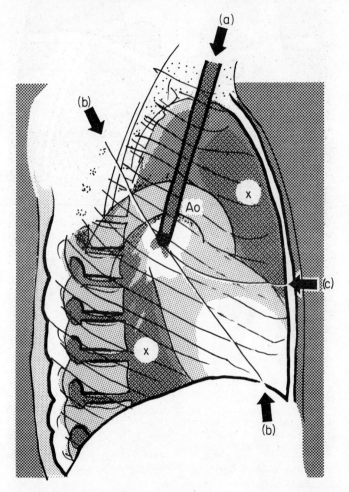

Fig. 7.2. *Diagram of chest X-ray* (*lateral view*
(a) Trachea. Ao: aorta. (b) Oblique fissure. (c) Horizontal fissure. It is useful to note that in a normal lateral view the radiodensity of the lung field above and in front of the cardiac shadow is about the same as that below and behind (x).

(net-like) or nodular pattern. Advanced interstitial fibrosis results in a honeycomb change which is apparent on the chest X-ray as diffuse

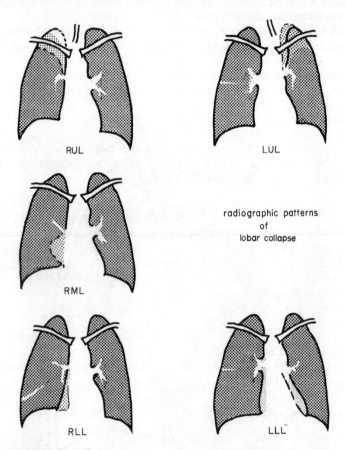

RUL   LUL

radiographic patterns
of
lobar collapse

RML

RLL   LLL

Fig. 7.3. *Lobar collapse*
Collapsed lobes occupy a surprisingly small volume and are commonly over-looked on the chest X-ray. In the above diagram note the position of the dia-phragms in each case. Helpful information may be provided by the position of the trachea, the hilar vascular shadows and the horizontal fissure.

RUL—right upper lobe   LUL—left upper lobe
RML—right middle lobe   LLL—left lower lobe
RLL—right lower lobe

opacification containing multiple circular translucencies a few millimetres in diameter.

Rounded shadows

Carcinoma of the lung is by far the commonest cause of rounded shadows in the lung; other causes include:
Metastatic tumour (? multiple)
Tuberculoma (? calcification)
Lung abscess (usually cavitates in time)
Pulmonary infarct (not usually round; tends to disappear)
Rare primary benign tumours (hamartoma, adenoma etc.)
Encysted interlobar effusion
Hydatid cyst (rare, ? hair-like outline)
Arteriovenous malformation (? adjacent vascular shadow).

Early thoracotomy is indicated in the case of rounded shadows without obvious cause as they are so often due to surgically curable carcinoma and diagnosis is commonly impossible by other means.

Miliary mottling

This term is used to describe the appearance produced by numerous minute opacities in the lung fields 1 to 3 mm in diameter (which may resemble millet seeds)—an appearance which may be caused by a very large number of pathological processes, some of the commoner causes being:
Miliary tuberculosis (see p. 91).
Pneumoconiosis (see p. 218).
Sarcoidosis (see p. 150).
Fibrosing alveolitis (p. 140).
Lymphangitis carcinomatosa (p. 179).
Pulmonary oedema (usually perihilar, transient and accompanied by larger fluffy shadows).

Mediastinal masses

Metastatic tumour or lymphomatous involvement of the mediastinal lymph nodes is the commonest cause of an abnormal mediastinal shadow but other masses may cast shadows and the particular site of the mass may give a clue to its cause (Fig. 7.4).

Special Techniques
Tomography

In this technique the film and the X-ray tube move in opposite directions along parallel axes pivoting about a point situated at the level of particular interest within the chest. The movement causes blurring of shadows except those situated in the plane of the pivotal point which remain fairly

sharply defined giving the effect of a cross-section at this level. Adjustment
of the apparatus allows several 'cuts' to be made in the region under
scrutiny. The technique may yield useful information in the investigation

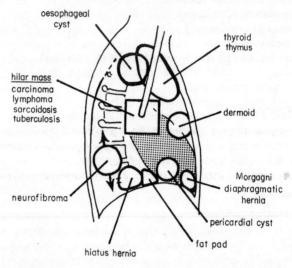

oesophageal
cyst

thyroid
thymus

hilar mass
carcinoma
lymphoma
sarcoidosis
tuberculosis

dermoid

Morgagni
diaphragmatic
hernia

neurofibroma

pericardial cyst

fat pad

hiatus hernia

Fig. 7.4. *Mediastinal masses.* Diagram of lateral view of the chest indicating
the sites favoured by some of the commoner mediastinal masses.

of pulmonary opacities particularly those situated near the hilum which
may be difficult to distinguish from vascular shadows. Tomography may
give a clearer outline of a pulmonary shadow, reveal the presence of calcification or cavitation not evident on a plain film and may demonstrate the
relationship between a shadow and adjacent bronchi and blood vessels.

Bronchography

A variety of techniques are employed for the introduction of an iodised
oily contrast medium into the trachea, generally under local anaesthesia.
It is an uncomfortable procedure. Immediately after instillation of about
20 ml (for one side) of the medium the patient is rolled and tipped into
lateral, supine, prone and head-down positions to fill the main bronchopulmonary segments. Oblique, posteroanterior and lateral views are taken.
Bronchography may be useful where it is important to confirm the presence or extent of bronchiectasis or in the investigation of bronchial
obstruction especially where this is beyond the range of the bronchoscope.
Bronchography should not be undertaken lightly—particularly in the
presence of asthma or severe respiratory disability.

Fluoroscopy ('Screening')

This is generally carried out with the aid of image-intensifying equipment. It permits movement of the lungs and diaphragms to be observed which may be important in the investigation of suspected diaphragmatic paralysis. Movement of the paralysed side is defective and if the patient sniffs the paralysed diaphragm will show paradoxical upward movement. Screening may also permit air-trapping in large localised areas of lung to be observed.

Pulmonary arteriography

Radio-opaque contrast material is injected into the pulmonary artery through a catheter which has been passed from a peripheral vein through the right side of the heart. The usual indications are (1) confirmation of pulmonary embolism and (2) identification of arteriovenous malformations

Lung scanning (see p. 192).

CHAPTER 8 · ACUTE RESPIRATORY INFECTION

Most acute respiratory infections are of viral origin. A variety of different viruses are responsible. Some viruses are regularly associated with a particular clinical pattern, most are capable of producing differing respiratory illnesses depending upon such factors as severity of infection, age of the patient and the presence of pre-existing disease.

Diagnosis in acute respiratory infections goes only so far as identification of the clinical pattern or the level of the respiratory tract which is principally affected. Pursuit of the actual organism is usually only carried out in severe disease in special centres or in the study of epidemiology.

PRINCIPAL PATTERNS

Common cold

Rhinorrhoea, nasal obstruction and variable conjunctivitis and epiphora are the main features sometimes associated with a scratchy mild pharyngitis.

Acute pharyngitis

The common 'sore throat' is more usually associated with fever and a variable degree of malaise. The throat and soft palate are reddened and the tonsils may be inflamed and swollen. After a day or two the tonsillar lymph nodes may be enlarged. In young people about 25–35 per cent of sore throats are due to infection by a haemolytic streptococcus; the proportion appears to be falling. Sore throat due to haemolytic streptococcus is indistinguishable from sore throat due to a virus.

Acute tracheo-bronchitis

Cough is the principal symptom. In the early stages it is irresistible, repetitive and unproductive. A barking sound is often produced by flapping vibrations of the inflamed posterior tracheal wall.

Audible wheezing and rhonchi are sometimes present. Reflex laryngeal spasm or actual oedema of the larynx may cause stridor. In young children inspiratory distress and croaking stridor may be prominent and the illness

72

is termed *croup*. Occasionally this produces dangerous acute respiratory failure.

Acute bronchiolitis

This term is used to describe lower airways inflammation occurring in babies mainly between one and six months of age. Initial upper respiratory tract symptoms, irritability and difficulty in feeding are followed by cough, wheezing and grunting respiratory distress with inspiratory rib recession accompanied by evidence of overinflation and, in severe cases, signs of respiratory failure. The baby is not usually pyrexial. The illness normally lasts 3–4 days and a rattly cough may last for 2–3 weeks. In severe cases respiratory distress may persist longer and it may be complicated by the development of bronchopneumonia.

Pneumonia

The term pneumonia infers inflammation of the lung parenchyma. Fever, tachypnoea sometimes with pleural pain and cyanosis together with clinical and radiological signs of consolidation are the main features. There may be profound systemic upset with delirium and circulatory collapse. (Pneumonia is discussed in more detail on p. 78.)

Influenza

The term influenza may be used by the lay public to describe almost any pyrexial illness but is generally used to describe an acute illness in which symptoms of malaise and particularly myalgia may be out of proportion to the upper respiratory tract symptoms and accompanying fever.

The patient is commonly prostrate and pyrexial for 3–4 days and may feel unwell and easily tired for a fortnight or so. Sometimes lethargy and depression develop and may persist over many weeks. The term influenza naturally acquires greater precision during the course of epidemics.

PRINCIPAL RESPIRATORY VIRUSES

Rhinoviruses

There are more than 90 different serotypes of this class of virus; identification and study are difficult. The incubation period is short and the commonest pattern of illness is the common cold. It is believed that rhinovirus may precipitate acute exacerbations of chronic bronchitis and may occasionally cause pneumonia in infancy.

Adenoviruses

There are about 30 different serotypes of adenovirus which may cause pharyngitis and conjunctivitis in adults, severe bronchitis in childhood and, rarely, severe pneumonia in infancy.

Respiratory syncytial virus

Respiratory syncytial virus is so called because it induces syncytial formation in tissue culture. This organism is the principal cause of bronchiolitis in infancy and is probably responsible for a proportion of cases of 'cot death'. Infection is commonest at about 3 months and is unusual before 1 month or later than 6 months, generally occurring in winter epidemics. Maternal IgG antibody does not confer immunity. Resistance to infection requires the development of specific IgA in the respiratory secretions. The virus may be identified rapidly by an immuno-fluorescent technique from nasopharyngeal or tracheal aspirates, by its isolation or by later serological changes. The organism may be associated with mild apyrexial upper respiratory tract infections in older individuals.

Influenza virus

Two main serological types are found, A and B. Influenza B causes mild recurrent outbreaks of influenza. There are several serological types but spontaneous antigenic variety is slight. Influenza A causes pandemic influenza. Spontaneous antigenic variation occurs from time to time resulting in rapid spread of the organism. Minor epidemics occur every winter and pandemics occur every 4–5 years or so. In epidemics patients with persisting chronic respiratory disease and the elderly are particularly at risk but occasional young adults may also suffer overwhelming infections sometimes complicated by influenzal or staphylococcal pneumonia, myocarditis and encephalitis.

Parainfluenza virus

There are four serotypes, types 1 and 3 being most frequently encountered. Epidemics occur which in the case of type 1 may show and alternate-year pattern. In adults this virus is associated with pharyngitis, laryngitis and tracheitis; hoarseness is a common feature. Fever is unusual. In children it causes croup (especially type 3). It may cause lower respiratory tract infections and a few cases of bronchiolitis are caused by it.

Coxsackie and ECHO viruses

These enteroviruses play a relatively minor role in acute respiratory infection. Well-documented outbreaks of acute mild respiratory illness due to Coxsackie A have been reported in closed communities amongst army recruits, students etc. Coxsackie B may cause pleurodynia (epidemic myalgia, Bornholm disease) characterised by fever and frighteningly severe lateralised chest pain on movement. This agent also causes pericarditis and rarely overwhelming myocarditis. Coxsackie A is known to cause herpangina-pharyngitis with vesicle formation.

Measles virus

Pneumonia and tracheobronchitis may complicate severe measles. It is difficult to distinguish the effects of virus infection from those of later bacterial invasion which may be protracted and lead to permanent bronchial damage. Measles may cause overwhelming pneumonia in children receiving treatment for leukaemia.

Epstein-Barr (EB) virus

This agent is known to cause infectious mononucleosis which commonly produces upper respiratory tract symptoms, principally pharyngitis and tonsillitis in addition to the other well-known features of the illness.

Other viruses

Herpes Simplex virus may occasionally affect the respiratory tract but is not commonly responsible for common syndromes of acute respiratory infection. Rarely it may cause pneumonia but almost always this is during the course of another illness or treatment which impairs immunological competence (leukaemia, immunosuppressive treatment). Cytomegalovirus may cause severe interstitial pneumonia under similar circumstances. During the course of chicken-pox the Varicella-Herpes Zoster virus may cause pneumonia which may leave specks of calcification which remain visible after chest X-ray. Chest pain due to pre-eruptive herpes zoster may cause diagnostic problems and sometimes herpes zoster is accompanied by diaphragmatic palsy.

Mycoplasma pneumoniae; Psittacosis/ornithosis
(see p. 83).

Treatment

Antibiotics have no effect upon the viruses described above but may occasionally be called for where bacteriological complications have developed.

Common cold

No treatment is generally required. Disabling epiphora, rhinorrhoea and nasal congestion may be ameliorated by an oral preparation containing pseudoephedrine.

Special risk cases

Patients who are thought to have had acute rheumatic fever or acute glomerulonephritis must receive penicillin for sore throats. Individuals with rheumatic fever should have continuous penicillin prophylaxis until they are aged at least 20. Penicillin may be given orally but prophylaxis may be more secure with monthly injections of a long-acting preparation.

Tracheo–bronchitis

Uncontrollable unproductive cough causing sleeplessness may merit treatment with a mild cough suppressant such as codeine linctus. Mixtures containing antihistamines are commonly found useful in children probably because of their sedative effects. If the sputum is frankly purulent and improvement is delayed an antibiotic such as amoxycillin, septrin or tetracycline may shorten recovery. Tetracycline should not be given in pregnancy or under the age of about 9 because of effects on teeth and bone. Croup in infants may be helped by maintaining a warm humid environment.

Bronchiolitis

Antibiotics have no effect. Treatment is directed towards presenting adequate hydration, oxygenation and feeding until spontaneous improvement occurs. Very occasionally progressive respiratory failure and exhaustion require the use of artificial ventilation—a specialist procedure not lightly undertaken. In severe deteriorating cases suspicion of staphylococcal superinfection may lead to administration of flucloxacillin.

Pneumonia (see p. 78)

Prophylaxis

Highly vulnerable individuals with advanced cardiac or respiratory disease may reduce the incidence of infection if they limit their contact with others by avoiding large gatherings etc. The common respiratory viruses are transmitted by droplet spread and it is almost impossible completely to prevent infection by isolation. Some protection against epidemic strains of influenza A is now possible with the use of attenuated live vaccines. Their use is normally limited to particularly susceptible individuals and injections given two to three months before the expected epidemic. The large number of antigenic varieties amongst the other common respiratory viruses has prevented wider application of vaccination in this field. During an epidemic, amelioration of an influenzal infection may be possible with the use of amantadine (used in the treatment of Parkinson's Disease) if treatment is started very promptly.

CHAPTER 9 · PNEUMONIA

Definition

Pneumonia is a general term used to denote inflammation of the gas-exchange region of the lung. Usually pneumonia is due to an infective agent but the term is also used to cover inflammation due to physical, chemical or allergic processes.

Bronchopneumonia/Lobar pneumonia

These terms have little clinical relevance but are nevertheless in widespread use. Bronchopneumonia is the name given to the most common pattern of pneumonia where there is patchy involvement of lung parenchyma, particularly in the lower zones. The term lobar pneumonia merely indicates that one or more lobes are uniformly affected by inflammation and consolidation with relative sparing of the remainder of the lungs. At one time lobar pneumonia was a common form and almost always due to the pneumococcus. Nowadays classical lobar pneumonia is rather uncommon and it is frequently not due to the pneumococcus.

Causative factors

Pneumonia may develop secondary to a breakdown of the normal defence processes of the respiratory tract—for example from failure to clear bronchial secretions due to impaired consciousness, age and weakness, overwhelming bronchial infection or lack of tissue resistance due to severe illness, malnutrition, alcoholism or immunosuppression due to disease or drugs etc. Localised pneumonia may be related to bronchial obstruction by foreign body or carcinoma or to infection of a pulmonary infarct, persisting bronchiectasis etc. On the other hand some agents appear to be able to produce pneumonia in previously normal individuals without obvious impairment of defence mechanisms.

In practice the clinical features of pneumonia give little guidance as to the nature of the agent responsible but the circumstances of the illness may give some clue (Fig. 9.1) (e.g. severe pneumonia in an epidemic of influenza A is commonly staphylococcal).

Pathology

The common feature of pneumonias is the presence of a cellular exudate

PNEUMONIA

Previously well infant
1. R.S.V.
2. Adenovirus and other viruses
3. Bacterial

Previously ill infant
1. Staphylococcus
2. *E. coli* and gram-negative bacteria
3. Viruses and opportunistic organisms

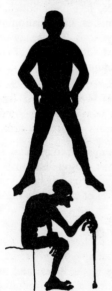

Children and previously fit adults
1. Viral
2. Pneumococcal
3. Mycoplasmal, psittacosis
Post-influenzal: Staphylococcal, strepto-
    coccal

*Previous respiratory illness. Elderly and
    debilitated*
1. Pneumococcal
2. Staphylococcal
3. Klebsiella
If no response to antibiotic treatment
    think of:
Tuberculosis
Mycoplasma pneumoniae
Carcinoma

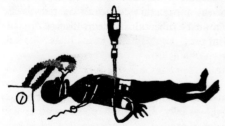

*In the course of major illness or
    during immunosuppression*
1. Staphylococcal
2. *Ps. aeruginosa* and other gram-
    negative organisms
3. Opportunistic organisms—
    Pneumocystis carinii. Cyto-
    megalovirus, Tuberculosis
4. Non-infective forms of
    pneumonia

Fig. 9.1. Some of the commoner organisms associated with pneumonia.
Age and previous health are important in assessing probable cause of pneumonia.

in the alveolar spaces. In secondary bacterial pneumonia suppuration may cause necrosis and damage to the lung architecture producing abscesses, cysts or damage to the respiratory bronchioles resulting in centrilobular emphysema. In lobar pneumonia due to pneumococcus and in some viral pneumonias resolution of the inflammatory intracellular exudate occurs, largely through the action of macrophages, and the lung tissue may return to its former state.

Clinical features

The severity of the illness and precise manner of presentation vary considerably. There is almost always malaise, fever and cough. There is commonly pleural pain and sometimes dyspnoea. Examination may reveal tachypnoea, tachycardia and sometimes cyanosis. There may be signs of consolidation (p. 41), sometimes associated with a degree of collapse or evidence of accompanying airways obstruction.

In severe pneumonia there may be severe prostration, delirium, jaundice, oliguria and peripheral circulatory failuer.

Management

Not all patients with pneumonia require admission to hospital, in fact the majority of cases is now managed at home. Hospitalisation is generally necessary in the very young, the very ill and in cases where domestic circumstances do not permit the necessary level of elementary nursing care.

Investigation

1. Chest radiology

A chest X-ray is important at some stage in the illness and as early as possible in the case of the severely ill patient requiring hospital admission. The extent and pattern of the changes on the chest X-ray is very variable but shadowing in at least one section of the lung field is virtually always seen. The chest X-ray may reveal important evidence of related disease (e.g. bronchial carcinoma, pulmonary tuberculosis, heart disease or signs suggesting pulmonary embolism etc.).

2. Sputum examination

Early examination of a gram-stained smear of sputum is important in seriously ill patients. This will usually distinguish pneumococcal and staphylococcal pneumonia from that due to gram-negative organisms such as E. coli, Ps. aeruginosa or Klebsiella pneumoniae which require different antibiotics. A Zeihl-Neelsen smear should not be omitted in case of tuberculosis.

3. Sputum culture

Culture of the sputum is always desirable and is very important in those critically ill, but treatment cannot be withheld until the results of culture are available. Interpretation of the results of sputum culture demands some caution—the organism retrieved may not be the causative agent particularly if antibiotics have already been given. Where there is good access to an interested laboratory specimens may be despatched for virological culture or immunofluorescence diagnosis.

BLOOD CULTURE

In severely ill patients it is often very helpful to carry out blood culture. Treatment appropriate to pathogenic organisms isolated by this means is imperative.

Pleural aspiration and lung aspiration

Culture of pleural fluid may provide helpful corroboration of the significance of sputum findings and lung aspiration with a fine needle may occasionally be justified in cases causing difficulty and grave concern.

Serological tests

Serological tests may allow a retrospective diagnosis of viral pneumonia if a rising antibody titre to one of the commoner viral agents can be demonstrated. This is rarely very helpful.

Treatment

General

The following measures are frequently necessary:
1 Encouragement of oral fluid intake to avoid dehydration.
2 Aspirin or paracetamol for severe fever, malaise and aching.
3 Stronger analgesics such as codeine, pentazocine or phenazocine for pleural pain. (Beware patients with previous airways obstruction if opiates are used, as respiratory failure may be precipitated.)

Severe illness

More severely ill patients may require:

I. OXYGEN

If cyanosis is present and respiratory drive is good oxygen should be given by nasal catheter or whatever method is best tolerated and in sufficient

concentration to relieve cyanosis. Care is again required if there is associated airways obstruction as the patient may have unsuspected chronic
respiratory failure (p. 160).

2. INTRAVENOUS FLUIDS
Severely ill patients with tachycardia, hypotension and a cool periphery
may have low plasma volumes reflected by a low central venous pressure.
Large volumes of saline or dextran may be required before central venous
pressure rises and adequate circulatory filling is restored.

3. CORTICOSTEROIDS
In very severely ill patients intravenous hydrocortisone is generally felt to
be beneficial although clear evidence in support of this is lacking.

Antibiotic and chemotherapy

1. PNEUMONIA IN PREVIOUSLY HEALTHY INDIVIDUALS
In this situation pneumonia is usually due to a virus or to the pneumococcus and this last organism is still generally sensitive to penicillin. Intramuscular benzyl penicillin should be given until there is obvious improvement when oral treatment with phenoxymethyl penicillin may be
substituted. In epidemics of influenza and where systemic effects are
dramatic, staphylococcal pneumonia should be suspected and treated with
flucloxacillin in addition to benzyl penicillin in case the organism is a peni-
cillinase-producer (as is increasingly the case).

2. PNEUMONIA COMPLICATING PRE-EXISTING DISEASE
Where a patient is alcoholic, debilitated or immunosuppressed or has
bronchiectasis, the possibility of a gram-negative organism should be
borne in mind. *Klebsiella pneumoniae* demands treatment with streptomycin 1 g twice daily in young adults (less in the aged) together with
co-trimoxazole. If *Ps. aeruginosa* is isolated and if the patient's condition
gives cause for concern or the blood culture is positive gentamycin and
carbenicillin should be given. This organism is often present in the sputum
of debilitated patients and its significance is then difficult to assess.

3. OVERWHELMING PNEUMONIA
In critically ill patients it may be necessary to treat blindly for possible
pneumococcal, staphylococcal, klebsiella or pseudomonas infection with
penicillin 2 mega units 6 hourly, flucloxacillin 500 mg 6 hourly, streptomycin and carbenicillin 4 g (all intravenously if there is shock) and
streptomycin and gentamycin intramuscularly.

Failure to respond

If the patient fails to respond to treatment the clinician should be alert to the possibility of underlying malignant disease, gram-negative infection, tuberculosis or mycoplasmal infection. The last generally shows prompt response to the introduction of tetracycline.

Complications

Pneumonia due to staphylococcus may produce cavitation and abscess formation fairly early in the course. Klebsiella pneumonia may be very slow to respond and commonly leads to abscess formation and to empyema.

Lobar collapse may complicate any pneumonia and bronchoscopy may be felt necessary if it persists in order to exclude intraluminal obstruction by carcinoma, foreign body or secretions. Bronchiectasis and localised pulmonary fibrosis may follow severe pneumonia.

Prognosis

The outlook in pneumococcal pneumonia occurring in previously well individuals is good and the mortality is of the order of 5 per cent. Klebsiella pneumonia still carries a mortality of about 45 per cent. Staphylococcal pneumonia is always serious even in previously well patients and the mortality is about 20 per cent. The most important factors affecting prognosis relate to host resistance. Factors such as advanced chronic cardiac or pulmonary disease, diabetes, alcoholism, malnutrition and immune incompetence secondary to disease or drugs all weigh heavily against a successful outcome.

Pneumonia caused by *Mycoplasma pneumoniae*
(Primary atypical pneumonia)

Mycoplasma pneumoniae (Eaton agent) belongs to a group of the smallest organisms capable of replication outside living cells. It may cause fever, sore throat, myringitis or pneumonia. It tends to attack in winter and occasionally causes local epidemics within families and closed communities. Children and young adults are the usual sufferers.

The pneumonia may be characterised by dramatic radiological shadowing usually in both lower lobes which may contrast with rather mild illness. Sometimes fever and symptoms of pneumonia may be very protracted if the cause is not recognised. Permanent damage or serious complications are rare.

Diagnosis

The diagnosis is usually suspected on clinical and radiological grounds, supported by a prompt response to tetracycline and confirmed by a rising titre of complement fixing antibody over 10 days. Cold agglutinins to type O human red cells are usually demonstrable in mycoplasma pneumonia.

Treatment

The organism is sensitive to tetracyclines and erythromycins.

Psittacosis/ornithosis

These names refer to the illness in man produced by *Chlamydia psittaci* which is a rickettsial type of organism transmitted from infected birds either of the psittacine type (parrots, parakeets, budgerigars) or others (e.g. pigeons).

Clinical features

The illness begins with a high swinging fever and dramatic prostration with headache, photophobia and sometimes delirium. There may be widespread myalgia and severe neck stiffness. This may lead to an initial diagnosis of meningitis. Splenomegaly may sometimes be detected. Attention is often not drawn to the chest until a chest X-ray is carried out although a persistent cough may be present. A few fine crepitations localised to one or more areas of the lungs are usually the only pulmonary signs. Enquiry usually reveals obvious contact with birds and occasionally the recent acquisition of a sick bird.

Investigations

The chest X-ray reveals some pulmonary shadowing which is usually rather undramatic and may be limited to one segment. Confirmation of the diagnosis is provided by demonstration of a rising titre of complement-fixing antibody.

Treatment

Tetracyclines produce prompt subsidence of fever and recovery is usually uneventful and complete.

Opportunistic pneumonias

A number of agents may produce pneumonia in circumstances in which there is severe depression of immunological responsiveness although they are otherwise incapable of causing it. These organisms are loosely termed 'opportunistic'.

Cytomegalovirus

This infection is most often seen in patients receiving large doses of corticosteroids and immunosuppressive drugs in the course of transplantation or during intensive treatment of leukaemias and lymphomas.

The presentation is as pneumonia, which is frequently severe and sometimes protracted, lasting many weeks. The chest X-ray tends to show nodular shadowing irregularly distributed in the lung fields. The diagnosis may be confirmed by rising antibody titres (immunosuppressives permitting), by isolation of the organism from lung aspirate, blood or urine. Lung biopsy may reveal typical inclusion bodies in the inflammatory intra alveolar cells. There is no effective treatment.

Pneumocystis carinii

This organism appears as minute oval bodies or cysts 5–10 μm in length and is probably related to the protozoa. It causes pneumonia in babies of a few months of age and in adults who are immunosuppressed. Breathlessness and tachypnoea are the main features, other physical signs are rarely helpful. Gas exchange becomes progressively impaired with progressive fall in transfer factor and ultimately cyanosis. The chest X-ray shows widespread mottling which is slowly progressive. The disease carries a high mortality partly related to the circumstances in which it arises. It may respond to treatment with pentamidine.

Aspiration pneumonia

Aspiration of acid stomach contents into the lungs can cause a very severe pneumonia accompanied by bronchial irritation and bronchoconstriction. Sometimes the picture is that of extensive pulmonary oedema which may develop after aspiration of quite small quantities of gastric contents (Mendelsohn's syndrome). Acute aspiration pneumonia usually occurs as a complication of states of impaired consciousness of whatever cause in which the normal protective reflexes are in abeyance.

Recurrent episodes of less severe aspiration pneumonia may occur in association with hiatus hernia, oesophageal stricture and diverticulae, weakness of the bulbar muscles, epilepsy etc. The episodes tend most frequently to affect the posterior segments of the right lung. Abscess formation is common. There may be very little to indicate the cause of the episodes of pneumonia.

Lipoid pneumonia

This is a special form of aspiration pneumonia due to the repeated un-witting inhalation of animal or mineral oils used medicinally (usually as laxatives or nose-drops; liquid paraffin is the commonest culprit). The inhaled oil causes patchy areas of pneumonia and collapse which may be widespread or localised, varying or relatively constant. Granulomatous lesions may develop which can mimic carcinoma. Cough is almost always present but there may be few other clues to suggest pulmonary disease. The diagnosis may be suspected when a chest X-ray reveals bizarre opacities in a moderately ill elderly individual who is found to be using an oily preparation. Microscopic examination of the sputum (or sometimes of biopsy material) shows 'foamy' macrophages which contain abundant globules of oil.

CHAPTER 10 · TUBERCULOSIS

Tuberculosis is an infection due to *Mycobacterium tuberculosis* characterised by necrosis and granuloma formation. It most commonly affects the
lungs but may involve other isolated organs or be widespread.

Prevalence and mortality

A hundred years ago more than 30,000 persons died from tuberculosis in
the U.K. annually (about the same mortality rate as for bronchial carcinoma today). A steady fall in mortality has occurred since that time due
initially to improved nutrition and living conditions, later to improved
public health measures such as early identification and isolation and in the
last 30 years to the development of effective chemotherapy. Death from
tuberculosis is now rare in the U.K. occurring mainly in the elderly and
sometimes being unrecognised in life. Despite the dramatic fall in mortality, tuberculosis remains an important disease and the annual notifica-
tion rate for new cases is of the order of 20 per 100,000. The average age of
newly-notified cases is increasing steadily. In undeveloped countries the
disease is still responsible for a large mortality and the pattern of the disease
resembles that prevalent in developed countries some 50 years or so ago.

Pathology

The typical appearances comprise the tuberculous granuloma with central
necrosis which has a macroscopic 'cheesy' appearance (caseation) and
which in time commonly contains calcium salts (Fig. 10.1). Healing
lesions are generally accompanied by extensive fibrosis. The extent to
which proliferative changes, fibrosis or caseation predominate is probably
determined by the immunological status of the individual.

Evolution of the disease (Fig. 10.2)

Knowledge of the time-course of tuberculous infection comes from before
the days of effective chemotherapy; the disease is no longer seen to evolve
in the characteristic fashion in the U.K.

Primary tuberculosis

Source of infection

The disease is always acquired from an infected individual who is ex-

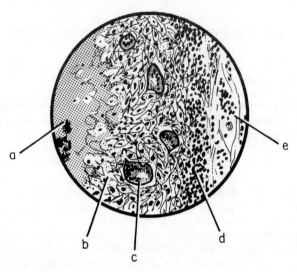

Fig. 10.1. Diagram of main histological features of tuberculous lesion. The centre of the lesion is to the left of the diagram. (a) Caseating central portion containing calcium deposits; (b) epithelioid cells; (c) giant cells of Langhans type; (d) lymphocytic infiltration of the outer layers; (e) fibrous tissue. The appearances vary considerably depending upon the age of the lesion, its situation and the degree of immunoreactivity of the host.

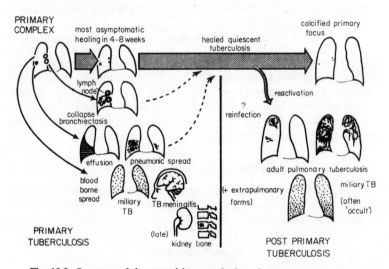

Fig. 10.2. *Summary of the natural history of tuberculosis*

creting bacteria; usually the contact is close and the exposure heavy. Less than 1 per cent of tuberculosis is bovine in origin in developed countries and this source will not be considered further here.

The primary complex

The primary complex comprises the reaction at the site of the initial infection together with that which develops in the regional lymph nodes. The commonest example is the primary pulmonary focus accompanied by tuberculous hilar adenopathy (Fig. 10.2). This develops within 4 weeks of first infection and usually its progress is limited and there are few, if any, symptoms. Occasionally erythema nodosum develops at this stage. Healing then takes place, the tuberculin test becomes positive, a degree of immunity to the turbercle bacillus is developed and the lymph nodes subside. The peripheral lung lesion becomes reduced to a small nodule which may calcify and be evident on the chest X-ray indefinitely (Gohn focus).

Progression of pulmonary primary complex

In children the lymph nodes may become much enlarged and cause pulmonary collapse by compressing lobar bronchi. Occasionally air-trapping causes overinflation of an obstructed lobe. Diffuse areas of radiological hazy opacification may be associated with lymph-node enlargement. This phenomenon is referred to as epituberculosis; it may be due to a parenchymal hypersensitivity reaction and it usually gradually subsides. In young adults the parenchymal pulmonary reaction may enlarge and cavitate with progressive pulmonary spread. Small parenchymal lesions may present with a pleural effusion identifiable by pleural biopsy.

SPREAD OF INFECTION
At any time in the course of tuberculous infection, spread may occur by several routes:

1. *Bronchial tree*
This leads to spread to other areas of lung or, via the sputum, to the larynx (causing ulceration) and gastrointestinal tract.

2. *Lymphatic system*
This leads to regional lymphadenopathy or ultimately indirectly to blood spread via the lymphatic duct causing miliary spread.

3. *Bloodstream*
Pulmonary veins draining pulmonary lesions may carry infective material

leading to remote spread of the disease particularly to bone, kidney, adrenal gland, brain and meninges.

Post-primary infection

This term refers to any development of tuberculosis beyond the first few weeks of a primary infection and after the development of hypersensitivity. It includes cases of reinfection and reactivated primary infection even when this occurs years later. Reactivation tends to occur in old age and in the course of illness or drug treatment which impairs immunological competence. The lungs are the most usual site of post-primary disease and the apices of the lungs are the commonest pulmonary site.

Clinical presentation

In developed countries the diagnosis is usually suggested by the finding of compatible changes on chest X-ray during investigation of patients with:
1 *Persistent cough and purulent sputum.*
2 *Haemoptysis.*
3 *Unresolved pneumonia.*
4 *Non-specific symptoms.* Investigation of patients of beyond middle age with fever, malaise and weight-loss may reveal tuberculosis. Immigrants from Asia and Africa may present unusual forms of tuberculosis with fever, malaise and splenomegaly associated with hilar or cervical gland enlargement.
5 *No symptoms.* Tuberculosis may be revealed during the course of routine examinations or by mass miniature radiography (MMR).

Physical signs

Almost any combination of physical signs may be found (e.g. consolidation, effusion, fibrosis, collapse). Quite often the signs are rather slight even in the presence of advanced pulmonary tuberculosis.

Radiological features (Fig. 10.3)

These override the physical signs in importance. A great variety of appearances is encountered including:
1 *Patchy solid lesions* of irregular shape tending to be localised to one lung or part of a lung or to the upper lobes.
2 *Cavitated solid lesions.*
3 *Streaky fibrosis.*
4 *Flecks of calcification.* Calcification is always suggestive of tuberculosis

but occurs in other conditions. All of these changes may be present together.

Other patterns which may be encountered include:

5 *Solitary round shadows.* Less than a quarter of these shadows are tuberculous and the majority of the remainder are of neoplastic origin.

6 *Hilar gland enlargement.* The combination of hilar enlargement and a solid lesion which may be cavitated tends to resemble bronchial carcinoma.

7 *Pleural effusion.*

8 *Pneumothorax.*

9 *Miliary mottling* (see below).

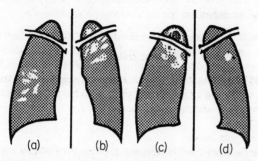

(a)   (b)   (c)   (d)

Fig. 10.3. *Radiographic appearances in pulmonary tuberculosis*
Tuberculosis can produce almost any form of pulmonary shadowing. Some common forms are indicated above. (a) Irregular mottled shadowing of any part of the lung especially (b) one or both apices. (c) Cavitation of an apical lesion is particularly suggestive but cavitation also occurs in carcinoma. (d) Solitary tuberculoma presenting as a 'coin' shadow. Calcification suggests tuberculosis but the diagnosis is generally only established at thoracotomy; the majority of such shadows is caused by carcinoma.

Miliary tuberculosis

This term refers to the widespread dissemination of tuberculosis usually with multiple (millet-seed size) nodules evident in the lung fields on the chest X-ray which is generally believed to follow entry of a large amount of infective material into the circulation either via the lymphatic system or the veins draining a local lesion. Formerly this variety of the disease was most usually seen following primary infection in children but it is now encountered more frequently in the older age groups. Usually the patient is ill, pyrexial and anorexic but occasionally individuals appear to be active and fairly well. A low-grade fever is the most constant of the non-specific features. Sometimes anaemia is the most obvious clinical feature and the blood picture may show abnormal cells suggesting a diagnosis of leukaemia. Occasionally these non-specific features are present without any miliary changes on the chest X-ray and the diagnosis may then be exceedingly difficult. Persisting fever in an elderly individual who is deteriorating may call for a therapeutic trial of specific antituberculous therapy even if attempts to isolate the tubercle bacillus have failed.

Diagnosis of tuberculosis

The combinations of clinical and radiological features described will often make a diagnosis of tuberculosis virtually certain but definitive diagnosis requires identification of the tubercle bacillus.

Sputum smear examination

Examination of a sputum smear stained by the Zeihl-Neelsen method by adequately trained individuals is a vital step in diagnosis. Identification of acid and alcohol-fast bacilli is presumptive evidence of tuberculosis and of infectivity (in an untreated case). Repeated sputum examinations are indicated where suspicion of tuberculosis is high.

Sputum culture

The tubercle bacillus can be cultured *in vitro* on Dover's medium. This takes between 4 and 7 weeks. Assessment of *in vitro* sensitivity to antituberculous drugs may take a further 3 weeks after positive identification.

Guinea-pig inoculation

This technique permits isolation of tubercle bacilli when they are present in very small numbers in the material. It is expensive and rarely required.

Biopsy

The diagnosis can sometimes be made from biopsy material and this is particularly the case with isolated pulmonary nodules which require thoracotomy, pleural effusion and tuberculous cervical adenopathy.

Tuberculin testing

After 3 weeks or so from the time of the initial infection hypersensitivity to a protein part of the tubercle bacillus is developed. Hypersensitivity can be detected by intradermal injection of a purified protein derivative (PPD) of cultured tubercle bacilli. The response is of the Type IV cell-mediated variety and takes the form of a raised area of induration and reddening of the skin. In the Mantoux test 0·1 ml of tuberculin solution is injected intradermally (not subcutaneously). The test is read at 48–72 hours. A positive result is indicated by redness and induration at least 10 mm in diameter (the lesion is slightly oedematous and can be located by palpation with the eyes shut). If active tuberculous infection is very likely 1 TU should be used otherwise 10 TU is normally employed and the test repeated with 100 TU if the result is negative.

HEAF TEST AND TINE TEST

The Heaf test and Tine test are widely used and convenient (Fig. 10.4). Positive mantoux 1:100 (10 TU) or less, Grade III Heaf test and a positive Tine test are roughly equivalent.

Significance

A positive tuberculin test merely indicates previous tuberculous infection. A negative test virtually excludes active tuberculosis (except in rare cases of overwhelming disease or severe immunosuppression). A weak reaction to tuberculin (less than 10 mm induration; Heaf Grades I to II) may be non-specific and indicate hypersensitivity to other mycobacteria. Weaker responses tend to be seen in the elderly. Exceptionally vigorous reactions suggest currently active disease. The principal role of tuberculin testing is epidemiological. Spontaneous conversion in childhood is presumed to indicate primary infection and treatment is usually advised. A source amongst adult contacts must be carefully sought. In the U.K. the policy of B.C.G. vaccination of tuberculin-negative children at about 14 years reduces the usefulness of the tuberculin test above this age.

Case detection

The great majority of new cases of tuberculosis are detected by chest X-ray examination of individuals in the high-risk groups already mentioned. Mass miniature radiography is important where the prevalence of tuberculosis is high. In the U.K. the yield of new cases from this source is now extremely small (less than 1 in 2,000 X-rays) and the service is being contracted.

MANAGEMENT OF TUBERCULOSIS

The management of tuberculosis may be summarised as follows:

1. Curative chemotherapy

This is achieved by ensuring that the patient receives
a   at least two drugs to which his organism is sensitive
b   in appropriate dosage
c   for long enough.

2. Prevention of spread of infection

a   Isolation of infective cases where appropriate.

b   Identification of contacts who may have become infected or who may be the source of the infection.

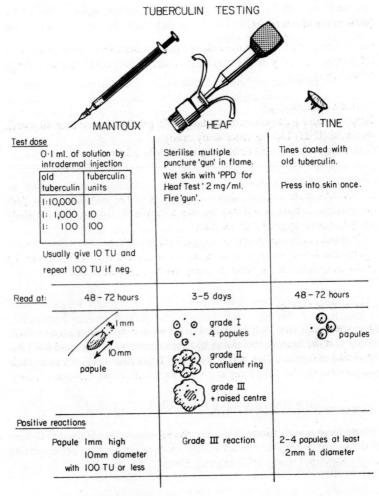

TUBERCULIN TESTING

	MANTOUX	HEAF	TINE
Test dose	0·1 ml. of solution by intradermal injection	Sterilise multiple puncture 'gun' in flame. Wet skin with 'PPD for Heaf Test' 2 mg/ml. Fire 'gun'.	Tines coated with old tuberculin. Press into skin once.
	old tuberculin 1:10,000 / 1: 1,000 / 1: 100 tuberculin units 1 / 10 / 100		
	Usually give 10 TU and repeat 100 TU if neg.		
Read at:	48–72 hours	3–5 days	48–72 hours
	1mm / 10mm / papule	grade I 4 papules / grade II confluent ring / grade III + raised centre	papules
Positive reactions	Papule 1mm high 10mm diameter with 100 TU or less	Grade III reaction	2–4 papules at least 2mm in diameter

Fig. 10.4. Tuberculin testing.

Curative chemotherapy

The aims stated above are simple but treatment nevertheless demands expertise and attention to detail and it should be supervised by doctors working as part of a health team with special experience of the problems involved.

Initial phase of treatment

Natural resistance to antituberculous drugs occurs and in the initial period before the sensitivity of the organism is known it is usual to give 3 drugs concurrently.

STANDARD REGIMEN
Streptomycin 1 g daily intramuscularly (0·75 g daily in those over 40 years).
Isoniazid (INH) 150 mg twice daily orally.
Para-aminosalicylic acid (PAS) 6 g twice daily orally.

RECENT MODIFICATIONS
1 Because of the high incidence of gastrointestinal symptoms with PAS treatment it is now customary to use ethambutol (25 mg per kg body weight once daily orally) in its place.
2 Because of discomfort and inconvenience of daily intramuscular strepto-mycin injections *Rifampicin* is being used increasingly (10 mg per kg orally once daily) in its stead. It is rapidly bactericidal in action.

Continuation therapy

Once the sensitivities of the organism are known only 2 drugs need be used. In the past the usual combination has been a mixture of PAS and INH but INH and ethambutol are better tolerated. Ethambutol is given as a single daily oral dose of about 15 mg/kg body weight during continuation therapy.

Minimal or probably inactive disease

Where there is only minimal disease, no organisms are obtained and there is doubt about whether the disease is in fact active. It may be reasonable to use ethambutol and INH together throughout.

Twice-weekly treatment

Where there is doubt about reliability of drug taking streptomycin and INH can be given twice weekly in slightly increased dose (together with pyridoxine to prevent INH neuropathy) under direct supervision of a nurse or health visitor.

Side-effects of the main drugs

STREPTOMYCIN
Deafness and vestibular toxicity especially in the aged and in renal impairment; usually permanent. Hypersensitivity in 10 per cent (see below).

P.A.S.
Nausea, anorexia and vomiting in up to 30 per cent. Hypersensitivity in 10 per cent.

INH
Peripheral neuritis in susceptible individuals and high doses (preventable and reversible with pyridoxine 1 mg orally with each dose). Generally well tolerated. Rarely INH may induce a reaction resembling lupus erythematosus.

ETHAMBUTOL
Generally well tolerated. Rarely optic neuritis leading to visual impairment (reversible).

RIFAMPICIN
Very rarely severe liver damage and thrombocytopaenia especially in those with high doses and in those with pre-existing liver disease. Rifampicin is excreted by the liver and is therefore useful in renal impairment.

HYPERSENSITIVITY
About 10 per cent of patients exhibit hypersensitivity to streptomycin or P.A.S. or both—developing fever and a rash. More severe manifestations with jaundice, lymphadenopathy and eosinophilia occasionally occur. The development of hypersensitivity was formerly managed by densitisation and corticosteroid therapy but nowadays a new antituberculous drug is substituted.

Failure of chemotherapy/drug resistance

This is almost always due to failure to take the prescribed treatment or to bacterial resistance (itself tending to develop through inadequate treatment). Smear-positive patients with resistant strains require isolation from the community. If the patient is not seriously ill treatment is usually withdrawn until a review of *in vitro* sensitivity to antituberculous drugs is available from a tuberculosis reference laboratory. Treatment is then recommenced with 3 drugs to which the organism is known to be sensitive.

Other antituberculous drugs

1 *Cycloserine*
2 *Pyrazinamide*
3 *Capreomycin; Kanamycin; Viomycin* (given intramuscularly)
4 *Ethionamide; Prothionamide*
These drugs are generally reserved for treatment of resistant tuberculosis by specialists.
5 *Thioacetazone* is an effective antituberculous drug given in a daily dose of 150 mg. It is cheap and is widely used in developing countries in place of P.A.S.

Duration of treatment

Early or minimal disease is generally treated for 1 year; advanced disease for 18 months. These times will probably be halved when adequate long-term experience of rifampicin has been gained.

Who needs hospitalisation?

Not all patients with tuberculosis need to be admitted to hospital and prolonged hospitalisation is rarely necessary except in frail elderly patients without supporting families. Hospitalisation is desirable in the case of

VERY ILL PATIENTS
Patients who are very ill and those whose domestic circumstances do not permit simple nursing measures to be undertaken at home.

SMEAR-POSITIVE PATIENTS
Patients with positive smear tests particularly where there are young children living in the same house. Adequate chemotherapy rapidly renders patients non-infective even though (especially with rifampicin) they may continue to produce positive sputum smears for weeks.

UNCO-OPERATIVE PATIENTS
Patients who are unco-operative and best managed in hospital during the initial phase of treatment and by supervised twice-weekly treatment afterwards.

See above.

Prophylaxis

B.C.G. VACCINATION

(Bacillus Calmette-Guérin) is a live attenuated strain of tuberculosis which confers a high degree of immunity. It is offered to all tuberculin-negative children at about 14 years in the U.K. It is given by intradermal injection. A local skin reaction is produced at about 4 weeks and there may be regional lymphadenopathy. The tuberculin test is positive after this time in successful 'takes'.

B.C.G. is given to babies and children in contact with known cases of tuberculosis.

CHEMOPROPHYLAXIS

Treatment is normally advised when positive tuberculin tests are encountered in children who have not received B.C.G. This is particularly important in adolescent girls because of the possibility of occult genital tuberculosis and subsequent sterility. A modified regimen may be adopted using INH alone in a single daily dose of 100 to 300 mg for a year. Prophylactic treatment may also be indicated in particular high-risk groups —for example patients with evidence of 'healed' tuberculosis who undergo treatment with steroid or other immunosuppressive drugs.

Atypical mycobacteria

About 1·5 per cent of pulmonary tuberculosis is due to opportunistic mycobacteria, the commonest of which is *M. kansasii*. The disease presents as indolent pulmonary tuberculosis and is identified in the laboratory. These bacteria are resistant to antituberculous therapy. A substantial proportion of patients with 'tuberculous' cervical lymphadenopathy harbour these organisms.

CHAPTER 11 · BRONCHIECTASIS AND CYSTIC FIBROSIS

BRONCHIECTASIS

Definition

Bronchiectasis is a state of dilatation of at least some of the bronchi. The bronchial wall is irreversibly damaged as a consequence of earlier inflammation and infection of the bronchus or neighbouring lung tissue, the normal transport of mucus is impaired, there is chronic local suppuration and the condition is characterised by cough and the regular production of large amounts of purulent sputum.

Prevalence

Most cases of bronchiectasis arise in childhood and as the population becomes replaced by individuals who have grown up in the antibiotic era the prevalence is falling and the mean age of those with established disease is increasing.

Pathological features

There is great variation in the extent and severity of bronchiectasis. The gross anatomical appearances are sometimes described as saccular, varicose or cylindrical but the actual form has little significance in terms of aetiology, course or management. The mucosal surface is always abnormal showing loss of cilitated epithelium, squamous metaplasia and heavy inflammatory cell infiltration. During infective exacerbations there may be sloughing, ulceration and abscess formation. The neighbouring lung is generally reduced in volume with patchy scarring and consolidation and may have been the site of earlier pneumonia. In severe cases the distal lung is replaced by fibrous tissue containing pus-filled cystic spaces.

Pathogenesis

The majority of cases follow severe bronchial and pneumonic infection in childhood. Severe whooping cough and measles are particularly prone to be followed by bronchiectasis. Bronchial obstruction by tuberculous

lymph nodes was formerly a common childhood cause of later bronchiectasis. Bronchial obstruction due to other causes such as carcinoma or
foreign body may lead to bronchiectasis in the collapsed lung distal to the
block. Proximal bronchiectasis may accompany allergic aspergillosis (p.
135). Bronchiectasis is generally present in congenitally atelectatic lobes.

Clinical features

The cardinal clinical feature of bronchiectasis is the frequent coughing up
of green sputum. There is considerable variation in severity:

Mild

Rattly cough and green sputum after colds only.
Changing position may produce sputum.
Occasionally small haemoptysis.
Patient generally very well; normal pulmonary function.
Normal chest X-ray.

Moderate

Rattly cough all the time.
Able to produce a specimen of sputum at any time—usually green, rarely
    mucoid. Occasional haemoptysis.
Patient or relatives may notice hallitosis.
Patient usually generally well, pulmonary function usually normal.
Rarely clubbing. Crepitations commonly audible.
Chest X-ray usually near-normal.

Severe

Very large volumes of khaki-coloured sputum.
Occasional pneumonic illness with haemoptysis and pleural pain.
Clubbing very common.
Particularly if associated with airways obstruction, dyspnoea, cyanosis and
    respiratory failure may develop.
Patient often generally unwell, off work frequently, may vomit during
    expectoration.
Pyogenic skin and ocular infections common.
Gram-negative bacteria commonly present in sputum.
At risk from pneumonia, septicaemia, remote abscess formation and
    (rarely) amyloidosis.
Widespread crepitations audible.
Chest X-ray may show increased bronchovascular markings and sometimes
    multiple cysts containing fluid levels.

Investigation

1. Sputum examination

Naked-eye inspection of the sputum is essential to confirm the patient's account. Direct smear examination and culture for tuberculosis should be included in the initial assessment. Bacteriological examination is often unhelpful despite the obvious purulence of the sputum. *Haemophilus influenzae* and staphylococci are commonly isolated but more often no pathogens are recovered. More advanced cases tend to harbour *Ps. aeruginosa* or klebsiella species.

2. Chest X-ray

This is necessary in order to exclude obvious localised lung disease but the appearances are often normal.

3. Bronchography

This investigation is expensive and uncomfortable and need not be carried out where the diagnosis is clear and management is satisfactory. It may be necessary where the diagnosis is in doubt—for example in the investigation of haemoptysis or recurrent regional collapse. It may also be necessary where management is unsatisfactory and there are grounds to suspect that the condition might be localised and treatable by resection.

Occasionally major saccular or varicose bronchiectasis is revealed but more usually the appearances are less dramatic and comprise: disturbance of the normal tapering pattern of part of the bronchial tree, abrupt failure to fill small bronchi in these areas and crowding of bronchi reflecting a degree of collapse in the part of the lung supplied (Fig. 11.1). The condition is generally patchy, basal and bilateral. Occasionally only one lobe is involved; left lower lobe and lingula are the commonest sites for localised disease.

Management

Management of bronchiectasis centres upon:
1   Postural drainage.
2   Antibiotic and chemotherapy.
3   (Very rarely) Surgical excision.

1. Postural drainage

The patient should be encouraged to 'tip' for at least 10 minutes up to 3 times daily regularly if by doing so additional sputum is produced. In mild cases this will apply for a week or two after colds and in severe cases

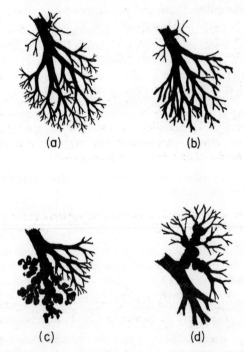

Fig. 11.1. *Bronchiectasis*
Diagram of appearances of bronchogram. (a, b and c left lower lobe; d, left upper lobe). (a) Normal. (b) Bronchiectasis. The normal graceful tapering of bronchi is lacking; bronchi are crowded and the finer peripheral branches do not fill. (c) Gross saccular bronchiectasis. (d) Proximal bronchiectasis with normal peripheral bronchi accompanying allergic aspergillosis.

it will be necessary indefinitely. Intelligent patients will discover the most productive position by trial and error. Usually a steep head-down position is most satisfactory.

2. Antibiotic and chemotherapy

WHEN?
Mild cases require an antibiotic after a cold and this will usually render the sputum mucoid. Moderately severe cases require an antibiotic after colds and more frequent courses of treatment may be worthwhile if this succeeds

in rendering the sputum clear for some weeks. If the sputum does not become clear then antibiotics should be reserved for acute exacerbations. In severe cases antibiotics may be worthwhile on a long-term basis if this appears to reduce the volume and purulence of the sputum and prevent pneumonic episodes. The long-term use of antibiotics carries some hazards (including candidiasis and the fostering of resistant strains of bacteria) and these must be weighed against the observed benefits.

WHICH ANTIBIOTIC?

Amoxycillin, tetracycline and cotrimoxazole are all effective in standard dosage. In long-term use the development of resistant strains can theoretically be discouraged by changing the antibiotic at regular (say monthly) intervals. Almost always cotrimoxazole will be found to be most effective whatever the results of bacteriological examination.

Severe illness

When a patient with bronchiectasis becomes severely ill the possibility of pneumonia or septicaemia from staphylococcus, pseudomonas or klebsiella should be considered.

Surgical excision

This is only very rarely appropriate because medical management is quite satisfactory in most cases and because the condition tends to be diffuse.

Prognosis

This is obviously related to the severity. The vast majority of patients are able to lead normal lives and have a life expectancy which is nearly normal. The outlook is much less certain in those with extensive lung destruction or airways obstruction.

CYSTIC FIBROSIS
(Fibrocystic disease of the pancreas; Mucoviscidosis)

This disease arises in about 1 in 3,000 live births from a genetic disturbance which affects all exocrine glands of the body and causes the secretions (including tears and sweat) to have an abnormally high sodium content.

Pancreatic lesion

The pancreas is the principal organ affected by the prime defect. The exocrine tissue atrophies and the ducts remain as dilated cysts—hence the name. Pancreatic failure results in malabsorption and steatorrhoea.

Pulmonary lesion

This takes the form of more or less severe bronchiectasis. The mechanism of its development is not certain. The mucus is not (as was once thought) excessively viscid but it is formed in excessive quantities from hypertrophied mucous glands. The serum of affected individuals has the capacity to inhibit ciliary activity and it seems possible that impaired ciliary action may be the principal factor in the initiation of the lung lesion—recurrent infection particularly by *Staphylococcus aureus* and *Ps. aeruginosa*, aided by accumulated secretions being largely responsible for subsequent bronchial damage. Malnutrition secondary to pancreatic failure probably lowers resistance to this bronchial infection.

Clinical features

Meconium ileus

A small proportion of cases present with this condition in the first few days of life.

Failure to thrive

About half of the total of new cases present in infancy or early childhood with respiratory infections; they are found to be small and malnourished with steatorrhoea. The remainder may develop almost normally and present with respiratory symptoms later in childhood.

Respiratory disease

The symptoms are those of bronchiectasis (p. 100). Clubbing tends to occur early. The pulmonary lesion tends to progress. The chest X-ray commonly shows a variety of abnormal features suggestive of fibrosis, nodular consolidation and cyst formation. These changes may already be established at the time of first diagnosis.

Diagnosis

The association of bronchiectasis and pancreatic failure makes the diagnosis very probable. In young children and infants the diagnosis can be confirmed by performing a sweat test and finding an increased concentration of sodium of greater than 70 mEq/1. The sweat test becomes unreliable in adolescence. It may be difficult to confirm the diagnosis beyond this age other than by demonstrating the association of bronchiectasis and pancreatic failure (for example using Bouchier's test). Sexual maturation is delayed and incomplete. A factor present in the serum is capable of producing a characteristic inhibitory effect upon fibroblasts growing in tissue culture and this may be used to provide support for the diagnosis.

Inheritance

Affected individuals are homozygous for the cystic fibrosis gene which is recessive and probably present in about 1 in 20 caucasians. Both parents are carriers and a quarter of the sibs of an affected individual would be expected to have the disease and half would be expected to be carriers of the gene. Carriers cannot yet be reliably identified. Affected individuals are generally sterile.

Management

Treatment is based upon maintaining an optimal nutritional status to help the natural resistance to infection and upon control of bacterial respiratory infection when it occurs. Parents and older patients require a good deal of regular medical and emotional support.

Pancreatin

This is taken in the form of granules or tablets before meals; the dose depending upon age and clinical response.

Replacement diet

In recent years impressive results have been obtained using a diet which is designed to be well absorbed without predigestion. The protein is provided as beef hydrolysate, the fat as medium-chain triglyceride (corn oil or margarine) and the calories are provided by a polymerised polysaccharide which obviates some of the problems associated with the consumption of large amounts of glucose. To these basic ingredients are added vitamin and mineral supplements. The diet is not very palatable but it may be tolerated if it is introduced at a sufficiently young age.

Pulmonary disease

The management is essentially that of bronchiectasis (p. 101). Chloramphenicol may be employed in very severe infections. Some workers favour the long-term use of flucloxacillin as a prophylactic against damaging staphylococcal infections. There is no convincing evidence that mucolytic agents or special measures to maintain high ambient humidity are of definite benefit.

Prognosis

Until recently survival beyond the mid 'teens was rare. Most children still die before this age but survival into the mid-twenties is being regularly recorded. The management and support of young adults chronic ill-health and alarming relapses may be particularly demanding. Death occurs from respiratory failure or in the course of overwhelming pneumonia or septicaemia.

CHAPTER 12 · LUNG ABSCESS

This term is customarily reserved for localised suppurative lesions of the lung parenchyma which are not obviously due to tuberculosis or other specific infections.

Aetiology

I. ASPIRATION

This is the commonest cause of lung abscess. Inhalation of food, vomitus, sputum or other material is particularly likely to occur in association with:

a States of impaired consciousness
b Alcoholism
c Incompetence of the larynx due to paralysis or sensory impairment (Myasthenia gravis, bulbar palsy, local anaesthesia etc.)
d Oesophageal obstruction
e Persistent vomiting
f Severe bronchiectasis
g Infection in the mouth or sinuses (particularly dental sepsis in the elderly).

2. BRONCHIAL OBSTRUCTION

Partial or complete bronchial obstruction leads to retention of sputum and subsequent pyogenic infection. Common examples are bronchial carcinoma and foreign body (especially peanuts and extracted teeth).

3. POST-PNEUMONIC

The centre of an area of destructive pneumonia may break down to form a lung abscess particularly when the pneumonia is due to *Staphylococcus aureus* or *Klebsiella pneumoniae*.

4. TUMOUR

Cavitation is quite common in bronchial carcinoma and this results in what is effectively a lung abscess lined with tumour tissue.

5. EMBOLIC INFECTION

This may result from secondary infection of a pulmonary infarct or from embolisation of infected material from other sites of sepsis in the body or from contaminated intravenous infusion fluids and catheters. Intravenous injection of unsterilised material by drug addicts is especially likely to cause lung abscesses.

6. OTHER CAUSES
Trauma to the lung may rarely cause a haematoma which may become infected. An amoebic abscess may develop in the right lower lobe following trans-diaphragmatic spread from an amoebic liver abscess.

Clinical features

Fever and obvious systemic upset are present at least in the initial stages and a leucocytosis is almost invariable. Later when the abscess opens into a bronchus there may be a cough with expectoration of large amounts of foul material which is variably bloodstained at first and later brown or green. Fever and malaise may recede as the abscess becomes chronic.

Investigations

CHEST X-RAY
The diagnosis of lung abscess is almost always confirmed by the chest X-ray which shows one or more round lesions of almost any size which with time cavitate and may contain fluid levels. Abscesses due to inhalation most commonly develop in the apical segments of the lower lobes (especially the right) and the lateral and posterior parts of the upper lobes (especially the right).

SPUTUM
Culture may yield *Staphylococcus aureus* or other common respiratory pathogens. Anaerobic bacteria may predominate in foul sputum which commonly yields no growth on standard culture. The tubercle bacillus must always be sought. Cytological examination for malignant cells is unrewarding when sputum is largely pus.

BRONCHOSCOPY
When carcinoma or a foreign body is suspected bronchoscopy may be relevant.

Diagnosis

Most lung abscesses develop during the course of serious disease and the mechanism of their causation may be evident. Thoracotomy may be necessary to exclude a cavitated carcinoma where such evidence is lacking or where the abscess increases in size. If a cavitated abscess is due to tuberculosis the sputum almost invariably contains acid-fast bacilli on direct smear.

Management

Management comprises:
1 postural drainage;
2 antibiotic and chemotherapy;
3 (rarely) surgical excision or drainage.

I. POSTURAL DRAINAGE
The most satisfactory position will be evident from the radiological localisation of the abscess.

2. ANTIBIOTIC AND CHEMOTHERAPY
In the initial phase of acute illness therapy will be guided by bacteriological examination of the sputum and the results of blood culture. Staphylococcus pseudomonas and klebsiella will require special measures (p. 82). Later penicillin in large doses orally, perhaps with the addition of probenicid to block renal excretion, will generally allow gradual healing. When the patient is no longer seriously ill there is less call to treat gram-negative organisms recovered from the sputum as they are unlikely to be responsible for the persistence of the abscess. It is desirable to add cotrimoxazole if *Haemophilus influenzae* is prominent or flucloxacillin if *Staphylococcus aureus* is regularly recovered. The great majority of lung abscesses heal with medical treatment but this commonly takes many weeks.

3. SURGICAL TREATMENT
Surgical excision is only occasionally required except in the case of suspected carcinoma or where healing is delayed beyond about four months. Occasionally complications such as empyema or bronchopleural fistula require surgical intervention.

CHAPTER 13 · ASTHMA AND ALLERGIC DISORDERS OF THE LUNG

CLASSIFICATION OF HYPERSENSITIVITY REACTIONS

The classification introduced by Gell & Coombs (1958) is still very useful.

Type I

The antibody involved is principally of IgE class. It becomes fixed in certain tissues and particularly to the walls of mast cells. Challenge with specific antigen causes an alteration of the cell wall which permits the escape of histamine and certain other locally active substances which are collectively known as mediators. The effects of challenge by the antigen are prompt and Type I is sometimes referred to as 'immediate' hypersensitivity. This type of reaction is involved in anaphylactic responses and in extrinsic asthma.

Type II

In this form of hypersensitivity the antibody involved is fixed to the surface of circulating blood elements and the reaction takes place intravascularly (e.g. transfusion reaction). Type II reactions are not known to be of importance in respiratory disease.

Type III

The antibody involved is of IgG class and circulates in the serum and permeates the connective tissue when there is local inflammation. When antibody and specific antigen come together in a tissue they combine to form immune complexes which activate complement to set up a tissue-damaging local reaction mediated by leucocytes. This sequence of events takes some hours to evolve and Type III reactions are sometimes referred to as 'delayed' hypersensitivity. Some IgG can be demonstrated *in vitro* by formation of a precipitate with specific antigen. Antibodies of this type are known as precipitins.

Type IV

In this category the immune response is mediated by the action of lymphocytes rather than by antibody. The best example of this form of response is the tuberculin reaction. It takes two to three days to evolve. The behaviour of sensitised lymphocytes is the subject of intensive research. There is some evidence that cell-mediated (Type IV) hypersensitivity may play some part in asthma and allergic rhinitis but the nature and significance of this involvement is poorly understood.

Types I and III are established as being of some importance in respiratory disease.

ASTHMA

Definition

Asthma is a disease characterised by variable dyspnoea due to widespread narrowing of the peripheral airways in the lungs, varying in severity over short periods of time, either spontaneously or as a result of treatment (Ciba 1959).

Extrinsic/intrinsic asthma

Much emphasis has been laid upon the distinction between extrinsic and intrinsic asthma. In practice the distinction is rather blurred and of limited value. In extrinsic asthma the identity of the external allergen is known or strongly suspected on the evidence provided by the patient's history or response to skin-testing. In intrinsic asthma such evidence is lacking.

Atopy

IgE (tissue-fixed, immediate reacting antibody, also called reagin) is normally produced in very small amounts and only in response to substantial exposure to an external allergen. Certain individuals possess a constitutional tendency to produce important amounts of IgE following mere trivial exposure to everyday antigens. Such individuals are referred to as atopic and they tend to exhibit asthma, hay fever and other forms of allergic rhinitis, urticaria and eczema. Usually the atopic diathesis is evident from an early age.

Control of bronchial muscle tone

CYCLIC AMP

Cyclic adenosine monophosphate (cyclic AMP) is present within cells throughout the body and appears to be the principal factor controlling many different specialist functions. There is now a good deal of evidence to suggest that the tone of bronchial smooth muscle is mainly controlled by the intracellular level of cyclic AMP. Increased levels of cyclic AMP are associated with bronchodilatation and decreased levels with broncho-constriction. The level of cyclic AMP is itself regulated by the effect of transmitter substances acting at specific receptor sites on the cell wall. Cyclic AMP is degraded by an enzyme, phosphodiesterase, and sub-stances which inhibit this enzyme (e.g. theophylline) increase the level of cyclic AMP and act as bronchodilators.

AUTONOMIC NERVOUS SYSTEM
Stimulation of β-adrenergic receptors on bronchial smooth muscle causes an increase in cyclic AMP and bronchodilatation. Stimulation of α-adrenergic receptors results in reduction of cyclic AMP and broncho-constriction. Cholinergic receptors are also present in bronchial muscle and vagal parasympathetic stimulation causes bronchoconstriction, per-haps by altering intracellular levels of another nucleotide (cyclic GMP). Other receptors probably exist which are specific for other substances released locally in the course of immediate or delayed hypersensitivity reactions.

Mechanism of the asthmatic response

A schematic representation of some of the factors believed to be important in the evolution of the asthmatic response is shown in Fig. 13.1. The mechanism of asthma is the subject of much research and even this ab-breviated version will probably require modification with time.

1 IgE is produced by lymphoid tissue in response to the extrinsic allergen. IgE becomes fixed to mast cells in the bronchial walls.

2 Exposure to further allergen results in an antigen-antibody reaction occurring on the surface of the mast cell which produces a profound effect upon the permeability of the cell wall.

3 This results in the liberation of mediator substances stored in granules within the mast cell.

4 Mediators include: histamine, slow-reacting substance of anaphylaxis (SRS-A) which produces prolonged bronchoconstriction, eosinophil chemotactic factor (ECF-A), bradykinin and others.

5 The mediators react at specific receptor sites on smooth muscle cell membranes and this is followed by reduced intracellular levels of cyclic AMP and bronchoconstriction.

6 Mediators also cause alteration in capillary permeability.

7 This may result in the entry of IgG and leucocytes into the bronchial connective tissue. A Type III delayed complement-fixing reaction may then occur leading to leucocyte damage, release of lysosomes, local tissue dam-age and release of prostaglandins and other mediators.

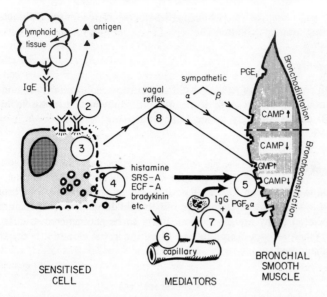

Fig. 13.1. Some of the factors involved in the evolution of the asthmatic reaction. The numerals are referred to in the text.
ECF–A, Eosinophil chemotactic factor.
PGE₁, Prostaglandin E₁—bronchodilator in action.
PGF₂∝, Prostaglandin F₂∝—markedly bronchoconstrictor in action in asthma
SRS–A, Slow-reacting substance of anaphylaxis.

8 Vagal nerve endings may be irritated by mediators, local inflammation leading to a reflex parasympathetic bronchoconstrictor response.

Pathological features

In fatal cases of asthma the main changes are found in the bronchial wall:
1 Eosinophil infiltration.
2 Increase in number of goblet cells.
3 Plugging of the bronchi with viscid mucus containing eosinophils.
4 Thickening of the epithelial basement membrane.
5 Possibly bronchial muscle hypertrophy.
    The lungs are overinflated but otherwise normal. Eosinophilia of the bronchial wall, sputum and sometimes of the blood is characteristic of asthma but the function of the eosinophil remains obscure.

Prevalence

Asthma is common. It is estimated that perhaps 5 per cent of the population has recognisable asthma in the course of a lifetime. Prevalence is greatest amongst children.

Mortality

Until comparatively recently asthma was regarded as a fairly minor complaint which did not cause death. Asthma is, however, responsible for over 1,000 deaths annually in the U.K. and many of these occur in young people.

Age of onset

Asthma may occur for the first time *at any age*. Males predominate in childhood and females in later life. In childhood extrinsic factors and associated atopy are much more likely to be encountered than later in life. When asthma occurs for the first time in the elderly it is commonly misdiagnosed.

Clinical features

The main features are wheezing dyspnoea, cough and an increase in sputum volume and viscosity. Sometimes the patient describes a sensation of choking in the neck or of tightness in the chest rather than wheezing. Sometimes the cough is given more emphasis than wheezing particularly when it occurs at night.

Patterns of variability in asthma

THE ACUTE ATTACK

Distressing wheezing of more or less acute onset is the hallmark of asthma. The majority of patients have such attacks at some time and often refer to them as 'spasms'. Some patients with asthma do not have abrupt attacks and suffer more or less persistent symptoms.

The patient sits or stands bracing the shoulders on the knees or on the arms of a chair. The expression is one of preoccupation with the business of breathing, breath by breath. Inspiration is snatched and expiration prolonged: both are wheezy. Examination reveals overinflation of the chest, use of accessory muscles of respiration and marked recession of the lower part of the chest during inspiration. There is a tachycardia and usually pulsus paradoxicus; cyanosis may be present. Auscultation reveals universal inspiratory and expiratory rhonchi. Most attacks subside spontaneously in minutes but some are prolonged for hours despite treatment (see status asthmaticus, p. 131).

Unconsciousness is occasionally encountered in an acute attack. Sometimes this is brief and suggestive of cough syncope and sometimes actual asphyxia accompanied by impairment of venous return due to overinflation seems a more probable explanation. Attacks of unconsciousness should suggest severe asthma and inadequate treatment.

Sometimes an acute attack is completely unheralded in a completely symptom-free patient but more usually attacks occur on a background of less severe symptoms.

EXACERBATIONS OF INTERMITTENT ASTHMA
One of the commonest patterns is that of exacerbations lasting several days or a few weeks after upper respiratory infections with long periods of relative freedom from symptoms.

CHRONIC ASTHMA
Some patients have persistent symptoms which may be mild or severe. Virtually always there is a characteristic diurnal variability.

DIURNAL VARIATION
Diurnal variation in symptoms is one of the most important diagnostic features of asthma and it is seen in chronic asthma as well as during exacerbations. The characteristic pattern is illustrated in Fig. 13.2. The main elements are:

Morning tightness
The patient notices tightness and wheezing usually within seconds of waking and this takes minutes or hours to subside. Coughing exacerbates symptoms.

Nocturnal attacks
Attacks at night are also characteristic of asthma. The patient generally wakes between 2 and 3 a.m. with tightness, cough and wheezing dyspnoea. He may sit up or rise to sit by an open window. Nocturnal attacks may be prolonged or repeated. Such episodes are commonly misdiagnosed as 'paroxysmal nocturnal dyspnoea due to left ventricular failure'. One of the most useful features which distinguishes this last type of nocturnal attack is the lack of morning tightness.

SEASONAL VARIATION
Marked seasonal variation is characteristic of extrinsic asthma. In the U.K. aggravation of asthma in the months May–July is typical of grass-pollen sensitivity. Aggravation in the winter months is common and probably due to two factors—frequent upper respiratory tract infections

and house dust mite sensitivity. Patients with sensitivity to mould spores are generally worst in the autumn.

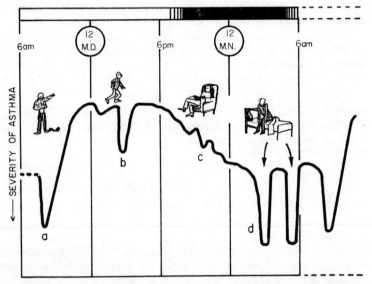

Fig. 13.2. *Diurnal variation in symptoms in asthma*
The most striking features are usually (a) chest tightness and wheezing dyspnoea on waking, improving during the morning and (d) nocturnal attacks. In addition there may be exercise-induced asthma (b) and worsening of symptoms whilst resting in the evening (c).

Trigger factors

A number of factors are known to aggravate asthma although they are not regarded as primary causes of the condition:

1 Exercise.
2 Non-specific irritants.
3 Infection.
4 External allergens.
5 Emotional factors.

EXERCISE-INDUCED ASTHMA
Severe exercise may provoke asthma especially in young subjects. Wheezing and tightness are experienced a minute or two after the end of exercise and are quite different from the hyperpnoea of the effort. If exercise is prolonged asthma may come on whilst it is still in progress. In some children exercise-induced wheezing is the only expression of asthma. The

mechanism of its production is uncertain. It is known that it is not related to the acidosis of extreme exercise and that different forms of exercise vary in their ability to induce an attack. Exercise-induced asthma can be blocked by prior medication with a β-adrenergic stimulant drug or disodium cromoglycate.

PROVOCATION BY NON-SPECIFIC IRRITANTS
Patients with asthma demonstrate hyper-reactivity to non-antigenic dusts, smoke, histamine and acetyl choline in concentrations which produce no detectable effect in normal individuals. Asthma may also be provoked by laughing, coughing and forced expiration. A vagally mediated reflex is probably important in the response to these non-antigenic stimuli.

PROVOCATION BY INFECTION
It is doubtful whether asthma is caused by specific allergy to common respiratory infective agents but it is certainly aggravated by viral and bacterial infections.

PROVOCATION BY EXTERNAL ALLERGENS
Allergy to foodstuffs is relatively uncommon but hypersensitivity to beer, wines, shellfish, eggs etc. is occasionally encountered. Airborne allergens may provoke asthma in minute quantities. In the U.K. the most common airborne allergens are grass pollen and house dust mite. Other pollens, moulds, animal danders etc. may also provoke asthma but these are numerically relatively unimportant.

Patients with grass-pollen sensitivity, as well as experiencing seasonal asthma, commonly have hay fever and are aware that proximity to grass particularly when newly cut is likely to induce symptoms. Camping is especially likely to provoke an exacerbation.

The house dust mite (*Dermatophagoides pteronyssinus*) and its close relative the kitchen mite (*Dermatophagoides culinae*) are minute 8-legged arthropods about 0·15 mm in length (Fig. 13.3). They are almost universally distributed and are responsible for the antigenic properties of house dust. *D. pteronyssinus* is found in highest concentration in the superficial layers of mattresses where it finds ideal requirements of warmth, moisture and its principal foodstuff—desquamated human skin scales. Subjects sensitive to asthma tend to suffer aggravation of their asthma:
1 at night—though not all nocturnal asthma is due to house dust
2 during bed-making and household cleaning
3 at week-ends (but excessive smoking, beer and wines may cause aggravation at this time).
4 in the early winter.

PROVOCATION BY EMOTIONAL DISTURBANCE

The relationship between psychogenic factors and asthma is complex but the following points may be made:

1 Severe asthma is frightening and chronic severe asthma is, in addition, depressing. It commonly results in chronic loss of sleep which aggravates symptoms of anxiety. In chronic childhood asthma in particular very great strains are put upon parents and child alike. Emotional disturbance in this situation is as likely to be a consequence of the asthma as it is to be the cause.

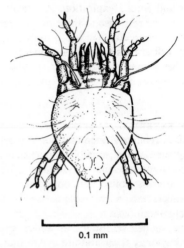

0.1 mm

Fig. 13.3. *Dermatophgoides pteronyssinus*—The house dust mite.

2 Psychogenic factors may undoubtedly aggravate the severity of established asthma and may provoke actual attacks. Anger, frustration and acute anxiety are particularly potent in this context.

3 It is widely believed that asthma is 'due to nerves' and this sometimes results in patients being rather unsympathetically treated by friends and relatives.

4 Some asthmatic patients are undoubtedly able to self-induce attacks. Usually this is brought about by repeated forced expiration near residual volume and this appears to produce reflex bronchoconstriction. This may sometimes be done more or less subconsciously to attract sympathy or avoid unpleasant tasks.

5 Patients with asthma are generally very appreciative of a straightforward 'organic' approach to the management of their disease. If asthma is adequately treated and if patients understand their treatment 'psychogenic factors' almost always subside.

Course

CHILDHOOD ASTHMA

The general trend is towards improvement. Perhaps three-quarters of children who have only very *occasional* symptoms related to upper respiratory infections will be free from attacks by the age of 15 or so. The outlook is less favourable in those with onset in infancy, those with a history of eczema and worse still in those with *continuous* symptoms.

ADULT ASTHMA

The outlook is similarly unpredictable. It is usually most helpful to suggest to patients that they will always have some tendency to asthma, that this may undergo spontaneous variation and that, with adequate attention to details of treatment, reasonable control of symptoms can be expected.

Skin-testing

Skin-testing is of limited value. It is undertaken for a variety of reasons:
1 To provide confirmation of immediate hypersensitivity to external allergens with a view to their subsequent exclusion so far as this is possible, or with a view to subsequent specific desensitisation.
2 To provide an indication of atopic status or to allow classification into extrinsic or intrinsic groups. This may not be of great importance to the individual patient but it may be relevant when comparing the results of treatment in different groups of patients.

PROCEDURE

There are two widely used methods.

1. *Intradermal method*

An extract of the antigen is injected intradermally using a tuberculin syringe and a fine needle raising a wheal about 3 mm in diameter. This method may reveal immediate and delayed reactions but tends to produce a high incidence of positive results of doubtful significance. In very allergic individuals severe local reactions, asthma or even anaphylaxis may be induced.

2. *Modified prick skin test*

A drop of each solution to be tested is placed upon the skin and a prick made by the method illustrated in Fig. 13.4. There are fewer false positive results with this method and the results correlate well with circulating levels of specific IgE. The quantity of antigen introduced is minute and the method is safe. It is much more convenient in practice than the intradermal method. Delayed responses are almost never seen.

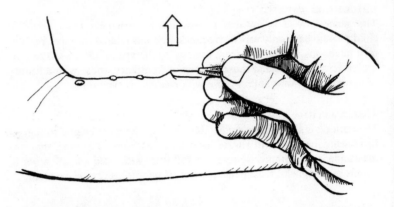

Fig. 13.4. *Modified prick skin test*
Drops of antigen extracts and antigen-free control solution are placed on the flexor surface of the forearm. Each drop is pricked with a fine needle. The needle is held parallel to the skin surface, advanced slightly and a tiny fold of skin lifted briefly as shown. Deep stabs and bleeding should be avoided. Wheal and flare are measured after 10 to 20 minutes. Fine disposable needles are adequate if cleaned and dried between each prick. Vigorous preparation of the skin is undesirable.

Note
Immediate skin-test responses are suppressed by antihistamines but not by steroid treatment. Delayed reactions are suppressed by steroid treatment. Patch-testing is not relevant to the assessment of immediate hypersensitivity.

Physiological changes in asthma

1. Airways obstruction

A. REDUCTION OF FEV_1
FEV_1, vital capacity and FEV_1/VC ratio are reduced and there is reduction of peak expiratory flow rate.

B. PROLONGATION OF FORCED EXPIRATORY TIME
This is generally evident even in mild cases with only slight reduction of peak expiratory flow rate or FEV_1/VC ratio.

C. OVERINFLATION

This may be evident clinically and reflected by increase in total lung capacity, functional residual capacity and residual volume.

D. REVERSIBILITY

Airways obstruction in asthma is often referred to as 'reversible' by bronchodilators. In fact airways obstruction is usually only partly reversible by a bronchodilator aerosol and the degree of reversibility tends to vary from time to time and between individuals (Fig. 13.5).

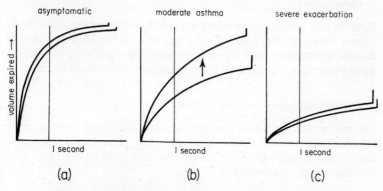

Fig. 13.5. '*Reversibility*' *of airways obstruction.*
Forced expiratory spirograms obtained from a patient with asthma on three different occasions. The upper of the two tracings was obtained some minutes after inhalation of a bronchodilator aerosol. (a) When asymptomatic, performance is almost normal and the aerosol produces little improvement. (b) During a moderate exacerbation of asthma the aerosol produces a major improvement. (c) During a severe exacerbation there is relative resistance to sympathomimetic treatment and there is little or no response to a bronchodilator aerosol.

Very large responses to bronchodilator aerosol such as shown in (b) are only encountered in patients with asthma but lesser responses are seen in asthma and also in patients with airways obstruction related to chronic bronchitis.

Trivial asthma

There may be little response to a bronchodilator as there is hardly any airways obstruction to reverse.

Moderate asthma

There may be a very large response to bronchodilator therapy.

Severe asthma

Little response is usually seen during severe exacerbations.

Although a very large reversible component (50 per cent increase in

FEV$_1$ for example) is seen only in asthma, lesser degrees of reversibility are seen both in asthma and in chronic non-specific airways obstruction associated with chronic bronchitis and are of little diagnostic importance.

2. Ventilation

In exacerbations hyperventilation is the rule. Only in critically severe exacerbations does the P_{CO_2} become elevated and this is a serious sign.

3. Oxygenation

Hypoxia is an almost inevitable accompaniment of severe exacerbations of asthma owing to the presence of areas of underventilation. Cyanosis denotes severe asthma and unless it is relieved rapidly (e.g. by intravenous aminophylline) it should be taken as an indication for hospitalisation.

4. Chronic respiratory failure in asthma

Chronic respiratory failure and cor pulmonale are rarely seen except in neglected, inadequately treated cases of asthma. Hypercapnia, congestive cardiac failure and right ventricular hypertrophy can all disappear after treatment with corticosteroids.

Management of asthma

It is very desirable that patients with frequent or persistent asthma should manage their own treatment as far as possible. For this to be successful (and safe) the patient must understand the use of each preparation employed and must have a plan of action prepared for unexpected changes in his condition. Just as in the management of diabetes, doctor and patient become involved jointly in an educational exercise which **takes time**—merely writing a prescription is not enough.

Control of extrinsic factors

Where specific allergens are identified they should obviously be avoided as far as possible. Complete avoidance of grass pollen is not possible but exposure can be reduced. In patients with regular seasonal grass-pollen asthma prophylactic treatment can be commenced at the beginning of the season on the first appearance of symptoms. It is equally difficult to avoid exposure to the house dust mite but the following measures sometimes help:
Daily airing of the bed
Frequent changing of bedclothes

Regular vacuum-cleaning of mattress and bedroom floor
Replacement of the mattress if particularly old
Trial of plastic pillow case.

It is rarely necessary to advise patients to move to a different house or climate or to dispose of pets or change employment on account of asthma unless the indications are particularly compelling and treatment is unsatisfactory.

DESENSITISATION

There is a limited place for desensitisation in the management of asthma. The treatment comprises repeated subcutaneous injections of weak extracts of specific allergen and it appears to act by inducing 'blocking antibody' of IgG type. The best results are obtained in patients with hay fever and a clear history of seasonal asthma together with strongly positive immediate skin reactions to grass pollen. Some treatment programmes involve weekly injections for up to 4 months but the trend is towards the use of fewer injections of delayed-release extracts given towards the end of the winter. Response to treatment is variable and difficult to assess because pollen exposure varies from year to year and because the patient will usually be receiving a number of other treatments concurrently. Sometimes improvement follows after several seasons of repeated desensitisation.

Recently improved extracts of house dust mite have been introduced and desensitisation to this antigen may prove more worthwhile than was the case with earlier preparations. Desensitisation to several allergens using a mixture of extracts is less likely to be successful than the use of a single antigen.

Review of available treatments

Bronchodilators

Frequent or persistently troublesome asthma should *not* normally be managed exclusively with bronchodilator drugs. They are most useful when asthma is mild or already well-controlled and they lose effectiveness during exacerbations.

BRONCHODILATOR AEROSOLS

Pressurised aerosols of β-adrenergic sympathetic stimulant drugs are extremely useful for the prompt relief of attacks of wheezing (Fig. 13.6). For example their use may abbreviate a nocturnal attack to a minute or two when it might otherwise last for half an hour or more and aerosol treatment is particularly effective in curtailing symptoms of 'morning tightness'.

Bronchodilator aerosols are best employed in putting the 'finishing touches' to asthma which is already well controlled. They should *not* be relied upon for the control of severe asthma when they are anyway ineffective. Salbutamol (Ventolin) and terbutaline (Bricanyl) are greatly preferable to isoprenaline as they are relatively selective β-2-sympathetic stimulants and

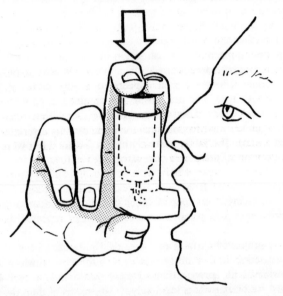

Fig. 13.6. *Pressurised aerosol in use.* The active preparation and an inert propellant gas solution are contained in a small pressurised canister which is housed in a plastic casing in an inverted position. Downward pressure on the base of the canister as shown releases a single standard 'puff' of aerosol. It makes little difference whether or not the lips are closely applied to the mouthpiece but it is absolutely essential that the 'puff' is synchronised with a vigorous inspiration.

cause little cardiac acceleration. They also have a longer action of up to 5 or more hours. The usual dose is 2 puffs as required up to a maximum of 3 hourly. If the patient is using a whole canister in less than 3 weeks this probably indicates the need for more intensive prophylactic treatment with cromoglycate or a steroid preparation (see below).

Cautionary note
During the early 1960s there was an alarming increase in the incidence of sudden death from asthma which seemed to parallel the increasing use of isoprenaline aerosols. Extensive publicity led to reduction in consumption and this was accompanied by a decline in mortality. The relationship

between isoprenaline aerosols and the sudden deaths was probably complex. The great majority of the sudden deaths were unexpected and occurred in patients who had received no steroid treatment and may have been attributable to the following causes:

1   Excessive use of isoprenaline may have caused ventricular tachyarrhythmias and sudden death from this cause.

2   Excessive use of isoprenaline aerosols has been shown to be capable of aggravating asthma. Some individuals develop 'rebound' bronchoconstriction after the initial bronchodilator effect and this may lead to escalating consumption.

3   Intensive use of isoprenaline aerosols probably disguised the severity of the asthma, allowing the patients to tolerate very severe asthma which might otherwise have been recognised as such and treated with steroids.

4   During an exacerbation of asthma bronchodilators may cause a *fall* in arterial oxygen tension (due to relaxation of pulmonary arterioles in underventilated zones). The fall is generally only a few mmHg and is probably only of importance in the very critically-placed patient.

The general public is now so aware of the dangers of aerosols that patients may be too frightened to use any aerosols. The use of aerosols and other inhalers is however very important and it is necessary to discuss the hazards fully with patients so that they may be seen in proper perspective.

ORAL BRONCHODILATOR DRUGS

A very large number of oral bronchodilator preparations is available. Like bronchodilator aerosols they are most useful when asthma is already reasonably well controlled. The patient should regard bronchodilator tablets as an 'optional extra' rather than essential treatment. Intermittent or regular use is reasonable if it produces clear benefit. Patients generally find that occasional use of a long-acting bronchodilator by aerosol has a prompt and lasting effect and they are unable to notice further improvement with the use of oral preparations.

The most widely used bronchodilator preparations contain ephedrine often in combination with a theophylline derivative and occasionally a small dose of barbiturate. Tremor and tachycardia are commonly troublesome. Salbutamol in a dose of 4 to 8 mg up to 6 hourly is as effective as any, has a long period of action and is very well tolerated.

Disodium cromoglycate (DSCG, Intal)

This substance has a **prophylactic action** and is administered by inhalation from a capsule in powder form using a special inhaler (Fig. 13.7). It is not a bronchodilator. It appears to act by stabilising the wall of the mast cell preventing the release of intracellular mediators (p. 112). If it is administered before challenge with an allergen it can completely block the asthmatic response which would otherwise occur. It is extremely valuable in mild recurrent or persistent asthma and young individuals with extrinsic asthma are particularly responsive.

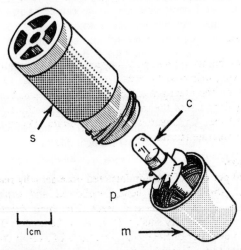

Fig. 13.7. Inhaler (Spinhaler, Fisons Pharmaceuticals Ltd) for administration of disodium cromoglycate. The mouthpiece (m) carries a central pin upon which a propeller (p) is free to rotate. The capsule containing disodium cromoglycate in a soluble powder base is fitted into a recess in the propeller. The two parts of the inhaler are screwed together and the capsule is pierced by two pins which are operated by a sliding sleeve (s). The patient first breathes out and then inspires vigorously through the inhaler causing the propeller to rotate. The powder is dispersed into the airstream. Two to four inhalations generally suffice to empty the capsule.

SOME PRACTICAL POINTS

1 It is essential to explain the prophylactic role of DSCG to patients and to stress the importance of **regular** treatment.

2 Patients should be warned not to expect a bronchodilator effect.

3 Coexistent active bronchial infection may prevent a response to DSCG.

4 There is no point in starting DSCG during an acute exacerbation unless it is a mild one. It will probably be ineffective in a severe episode and then rejected as useless by the patient. During a severe exacerbation steroid treatment may be necessary.

The usual dose is the contents of one capsule inhaled four times daily. Trial and error may show that optimal control is obtained with between one and eight capsules daily. Some patients are irritated by the inhalation which may produce cough and reflex wheezing. In these individuals it is appropriate to use a compound preparation which contains a small quantity of isoprenaline which abolishes this effect. Patients should not be started on the compound preparation without good reason as the bronchodilator effect of the isoprenaline may make it difficult to assess response to DSCG.

Steroid aerosols

The advent of highly topically-active steroids of inherently low glucocorticoid activity, delivered by pressurised aerosol (Fig. 13.6) has had a major impact on the management of bronchial asthma. Steroid aerosols now form the hinge-pin of the treatment of chronic asthma. Two preparations are available, beclomethasone dipropionate (Becotide) and betamethasone 17-valerate (Bextasol).

DISTRIBUTION
Only about 20 per cent of the administered dose actually reaches the respiratory tract, the remainder being swallowed and probably largely absorbed from the gastrointestinal tract. The high degree of topical activity however allows very small total doses to be used so that in normal use there is no evidence of the usual side effects of steroid therapy and no evidence of pituitary-adrenal suppression.

DOSAGE
The usual dosage is 2 puffs 4 times daily. Many patients are well controlled on as little as 2 puffs daily. Occasionally some advantage is achieved by increasing the dose to 4 puffs 4 times daily but improvement is not seen on higher doses and significant systemic absorption may occur (1 puff of beclomethasone dipropionate = 50 μg; 1 puff of betamethasone 17-valerate = 100 μg).

It is important to ensure that the patient can use the aerosol properly. Some coaching is commonly required and some elderly patients may never be able to inhale effectively.

As in the case of DSCG it is essential that the patient should understand the prophylactic role of treatment, the need for regular administration and the fact that no bronchodilator effect is to be expected. Improvement in chronic asthma is generally evident within a day or two and is often dramatic. Steroid aerosol treatment should not be used alone in a severe exacerbation; it may be ineffective because of excessive secretions or imperfect distribution and the patient may become prematurely disenchanted with the treatment.

FURTHER POINTS CONCERNING STEROID AEROSOL TREATMENT
1 Patients should not run out of aerosol or deterioration may be quite dramatic.

2   Severe exacerbations occurring in the course of aerosol treatment may require treatment with oral steroids. Patients with severe asthma should be taught to start treatment with prednisone themselves.

3   Particular care must be given to patients in whom regular oral steroid therapy has been successfully replaced by aerosol steroids. They may be at risk both from dramatic deterioration in their asthma and from hypoadrenal symptoms for many months after substitution.

SIDE EFFECTS

About 10 per cent of patients develop patches of candidal infection on the palate or pharynx although most do not complain of this. This complication is more common when high doses are used and it responds to treatment with nystatin or amphotericin lozenges. There is no evidence that candidal infestation extends below the larynx. There is no evidence that the connective tissue of the respiratory tract suffers from atrophy of the sort observed in skin exposed to high doses of topical steroid creams.

Oral steroid therapy

A. SHORT-TERM

Oral steroid therapy is indicated in all alarmingly progressive exacerbations of bronchial asthma—there is no call to wait until the patient is *in extremis*. Any patient sufficiently ill to require intravenous aminophylline probably requires oral steroid therapy—at least until the exacerbation subsides over a few days or until regular prophylactic therapy with DSCG or steroid aerosol can be established. Once a response to oral steroid administration is obvious the dose can be progressively reduced and often withdrawn within a week.

B. LONG-TERM

The need for long-term treatment usually becomes obvious when asthma fails to be *reasonably* controlled by other means and when short courses are required very frequently despite treatment with DSCG and steroid aerosols. It is very desirable that the patient should control his own dosage. He must understand the compromise which is being attempted between disabling asthma on the one hand and the risk of side effects on the other. The plan should always be to reduce the dose to the lowest level compatible with reasonable control of asthma. There should be no hesitation in promptly increasing the dose in the event of progressive deterioration over hours or days. Prednisone and prednisolone are the most widely used preparations and there is no good reason to use other corticosteroids. In 'titrating' the lowest tolerable dose 1 mg tablets are often useful used in combination with the standard 5 mg tablets.

Side effects

The general public in the U.K. is very aware that steroids produce side effects and it is common for patients with severe asthma to put themselves at some risk through failing to restart or increase the dose of steroid because of fear of the consequences. A common fear is that use of steroid treatment will lead to 'resistance' and gradually escalating requirements. There is no evidence that this tendency exists. Blatant over-indulgence in too high a dose is uncommon. In many patients worthwhile benefit is obtained with a regular dose of 5 to 7·5 mg of prednisone daily at which level serious side effects are not seen. At doses up to 12·5 mg daily some cushingoid redistribution of fat and facial fullness is seen. Most patients gain weight but this is capable of control by dietary restriction. At higher doses obvious cushingoid changes are seen and predisposed individuals may develop glucose intolerance, peptic ulceration etc. Only a very few severely incapacitated individuals can be shown to obtain worthwhile benefit from daily doses in excess of 20 mg daily of prednisone. Probably the most sinister complication is vertebral collapse from osteoporosis which is particularly likely to affect post-menopausal females.

REPLACEMENT OF ORAL STEROID THERAPY

In more than half of patients well controlled on 7·5 mg or less of prednisone daily the use of an aerosol steroid preparation will enable oral treatment to be withdrawn. In most of the remainder some reduction in oral treatment is possible. Withdrawal of regular oral steroid therapy should be gradual as there is some risk of hypoadrenal crisis which may accompany a dramatic relapse of asthma or some other intercurrent illness. Hypoadrenal symptoms may not be recognised as such; they may include: profound lethargy, anorexia, vomiting, diarrhoea, headache and muscular aching.

Where these features are encountered it may be necessary to withdraw steroids over a year or more. The use of ACTH or tetracosactrin does little to help this withdrawal as the failure is not merely adrenal but involves the pituitary-adrenal axis as a whole. The patient must be encouraged to endure mild withdrawal symptoms and to reduce the dose exceedingly slowly particularly over the last 5 mg of prednisone. A return of allergic rhinitis or eczema sometimes accompanies withdrawal of oral steroid treatment. It is sometimes safer to leave a patient on a small oral dose of prednisone if understanding is limited.

Antibiotics

Antibiotics have a relatively minor part to play in the management of asthma. It is difficult to be certain when active bronchial infection is playing an important part but the best guide is probably the production of yellow sputum. Bacteriological examination is not very helpful. If yellow sputum is produced it is reasonable to prescribe a 5-day course of cotrimoxazole, tetracycline or amoxicillin (but beware penicillin-sensitive individuals) as well as advising an increase in suppressive therapy which is usually indicated.

Asthma in childhood

Mild asthma tends to be aggravated by colds. At such times ephedrine at night may be all that is required. More persistent or recurrent asthma is often very responsive to DSCG which even children of 3 to 4 can be trained to use. More severe asthma may respond to steroid aerosol treatment in half the adult dosage.

SEVERE CHILDHOOD ASTHMA

An isolated severe exacerbation may be managed with a short course of oral prednisone.

Severe chronic asthma in childhood is sometimes not obvious. The usual marked fluctuations in severity and overt wheezing may be lacking and the parents and child may become accustomed to a limited level of activity. Stunting and chest deformity (Fig. 13.8) are indicative of severe asthma. As it may be difficult to judge the severity of asthma spirometry is very important. A small number of children are not adequately controlled by regular treatment with DSCG or aerosol steroids. In this situation the use of ACTH or tetracosactrin is preferable to long-term oral steroid treatment as growth suppression appears to be less. Injections are given 2 or 3 times weekly and the dose is maintained at the lowest tolerable level.

Asthma in pregnancy

Asthma usually poses no particular problems in pregnancy. Occasionally exacerbations occur in the first few weeks but the last 2 trimesters are often marked by unusually good control. It is common for exacerbations to occur 4 to 6 weeks after delivery.

Assessment of progress in chronic asthma

Because of the striking diurnal and day to day variation in the severity of asthma, spirometric measurements made at infrequent intervals may not be particularly helpful in assessing progress (Fig. 13.9). It is relevant to make a note of:

1 Number of nocturnal attacks (for example in a week).

2   The length of time taken for the chest to feel clear in the mornings.
3   Absence from work or school.
4   Consumption of bronchodilator preparations.
When assessing the effect of changes in treatment it is sometimes helpful
for the patient to use a peak flow meter or gauge at home making recordings twice or three times daily. Improvement is usually accompanied by
'ironing out' of the morning and sometimes evening troughs.

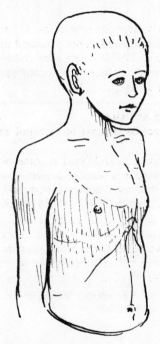

Fig. 13.8. *Chest deformity in childhood asthma*
The sternum is pushed forwards (pigeon-chest deformity) and there is a groove
approximately in the position of the sixth rib (Harrison's sulcus). Deformity
of the type shown is always indicative of severe asthma. It is to a considerable
extent reversible if asthma is treated adequately and sufficiently early.

Status asthmaticus

A severe, progressive, prolonged attack of immobilising asthma which is
unresponsive to bronchodilator preparations is termed status asthmaticus.
Treatment may be started in the home but hospitalisation is indicated.
Management is based upon giving large doses of corticosteroids and ensuring adequate oxygenation of the patient until the attack abates.

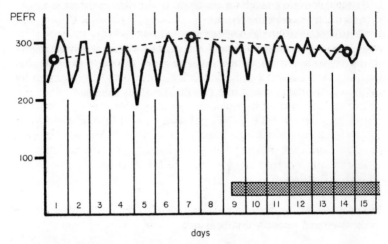

days

Fig. 13.9. *Fallibility of isolated ventilatory tests in asthma*
Solid line: Record of peak expiratory flow rate (PEFR) measured 4 times daily
The shaded area represents the start of new treatment (e.g. cromoglycate or
steroid aerosol). Typical diurnal variation is present over the first 9 days.
Thereafter there is progressive disappearance of the early morning 'trough'
although values obtained later in the day remain similar to those recorded
earlier.
Interrupted line: This line connects three isolated recordings of PEFR made
at three separate visits to a doctor. The doctor viewing only these results might
have been tempted to conclude that at the second visit there was some improvement and that there had been deterioration between the second and third
visits. The erroneous conclusion might have been that the new treatment was
ineffective. In this situation adequate questioning of the patient would almost
certainly lead to the clinician reaching the correct conclusion despite the
PEFR recordings he had obtained.

A. Initial treatment

I. STEROID THERAPY
Hydrocortisone (100 or 200 mg i.v.) should be given as soon as possible.
A large oral dose of prednisone should be given (20 mg 6 hourly until
improvement is obvious). If large doses of intravenous hydrocortisone are
continued hypokalaemia and weakness may be induced over 48 hours
or so.

2. BRONCHODILATOR THERAPY
Aminophylline 250 mg or 500 mg may be given by slow intravenous
injection up to 3 hourly initially and may produce partial relief of distress.
There is little to choose between an infusion and repeated slow injections.
An infusion preserves ready access for intravenous therapy in the event of

unexpected collapse and allows correction of dehydration which is usually present if the exacerbation has been protracted. Terbutaline (0·5 mg sub-cutaneously up to 3 hourly) may be used as an alternative to aminophylline. Although aerosol bronchodilators alone are relatively ineffective in this situation, when used in combination with an infusion of aminophylline they may exert a useful synergistic effect. If the patient is familiar with the use of a pressurised aerosol it is reasonable to use 2 puffs of salbutamol up to hourly if an effect is produced. Patients unable to use a pressurised aerosol may benefit from salbutamol administered intermittently by an oxygen mask incorporationg a small nebuliser. It is doubful whether more elaborate forms of bronchodilator nebulisation or hand-held positive pressure ventilators have any advantage in this situation.

3. REASSURANCE
The patient must be made to feel firstly that his desperate symptoms are understood and secondly that he is safe.

4. OXYGEN THERAPY
Hypoxia is usual in severe asthma and administration of oxygen using a mask which delivers a high concentration is appropriate and usually safe. Almost always the drive to breathe is well preserved; very occasionally exhausted patients who have endured a prolonged exacerbation may be in chronic respiratory failure and require controlled oxygen therapy (p. 168).

There is no place for the regular use of sedative drugs in the manage-ment of status asthmaticus. The patient in status asthmaticus needs every bit of respiratory drive he can muster.

B. Assessment phase

Once initial treatment is established a period of extreme vigilance follows. Progress may be assessed by observation of:

I. PULSE RATE

2. THE APPEARANCE OF THE PATIENT
Important information is provided by observing the patient's position in bed, the character of his breathing, facial expression and his own assess-ment of progress. The auscultatory signs are of little help—reduction in rhonchi may actually indicate deterioration.

3. ESTIMATION OF BLOOD GAS TENSIONS
When IPPV is being seriously considered this is of particular value. Even borderline elevation of the $P\text{co}_2$ is a serious sign—it means that the best efforts of the patient's respiratory drive result in inadequate ventilation. Cyanosis whilst breathing oxygen-enriched air is a particularly sinister sign and is usually a compelling argument for IPPV.

4. PULMONARY FUNCTION TESTS

The patient is almost always too distressed to undertake even the simplest spirometric tests until there has been substantial improvement; they are of little help.

C. Intermittent Positive Pressure Ventilation (IPPV)

INDICATIONS

IPPV is only rarely necessary, and is used when there is:

1 Inability to secure adequate oxygenation of the patient.

2 Exhaustion—as suggested by progressive tiredness, hopelessness and apathy accompanied by a rising P_{CO_2}, rising pulse rate and failure to produce sputum.

PURPOSE

The purpose is to ensure adequate oxygenation of the patient until the other therapeutic measures bring the attack to an end.

MEANS

1 Control of the patient's airway ensures that oxygen administration is continuous. It is possible to administer higher concentrations of oxygen by IPPV than by mask.

2 A minimum ventilation is secured. Some underventilation is acceptable.

3 The patient can be sedated and rested once the breathing is under control by IPPV.

4 Clearing of tenacious bronchial secretions can be assisted by suction—sometimes assisted by lavage with small quantities of warmed water or saline injected into the airway.

In practice IPPV is carried out by endotracheal intubation with sedation using drugs such as phenoperidine (a short-acting opiate derivative) and muscle relaxants. IPPV may be necessary for as little as a few hours or for more than a week.

D. Convalescence

Once improvement is obvious and sustained over 24 hours attention can be given to reduction of the dose of steroid and other drugs and to **education of the patient** in the management of his asthma. The patient can be discharged from hospital once he is mobile and he fully understands his treatment. There is no call to wait until oral steroid therapy has been withdrawn completely. It is preferable for the last 10 to 15 mg of prednisone to be withdrawn after discharge from hospital.

Prevention

Almost always status asthmaticus is preventable. Severe exacerbations are usually preceded by a period of gradual deterioration which should be the signal for the patient with severe asthma to start or increase oral steroid treatment. If this is done promptly, status asthmaticus is generally averted.

BRONCHOPULMONARY ASPERGILLOSIS

The clinical patterns of disease related to the ubiquitous mould *Aspergillus fumigatus* are illustrated in Fig. 13.10. In allergic aspergillosis both immediate and delayed responses are usually demonstrable by intradermal skin testing and by bronchial challenge (the latter is not part of routine diagnostic procedure). The recognition of allergic aspergillosis does not usually affect management; asthma is treated on its merits as outlined above. Desensitisation is not helpful and antifungal treatment is not yet very satisfactory. Steroid treatment either by mouth or aerosol is usually fairly effective.

Episodes of lobar collapse due to 'mucoid impaction' may be treated by bronchoscopy and bronchial lavage. Usually the collapse resolves spontaneously or with the help of steroid therapy.

Mycetomas have a characteristic radiographic appearance. They lie free within the cavity and there is a thin rim of radiolucency ('halo') surrounding the rounded mass. Mycetomas enlarge very slowly; some cause massive haemoptysis. Surgical removal is indicated if haemoptysis is threatening and lung function is good.

PULMONARY EOSINOPHILIA

This term is used to cover a variety of conditions in which radiological pulmonary shadowing is associated with a very high blood eosinophil count. The radiological shadows may be fluffy, wedge-shaped or reticulonodular in type.

1. Pulmonary eosinophilia with asthma

The majority of patients with fleeting isolated shadows and asthma have allergic aspergillosis and supporting evidence in the shape of skin test reactions, the presence of serum precipitins and regular recovery of the organism is commonly forthcoming. Other antigens (e.g. house dust mite) may be capable of inducing pulmonary eosinophilia. Sometimes no obvious association with an antigen can be found.

SYNOPSIS OF BRONCHO- PULMONARY ASPERGILLOSIS

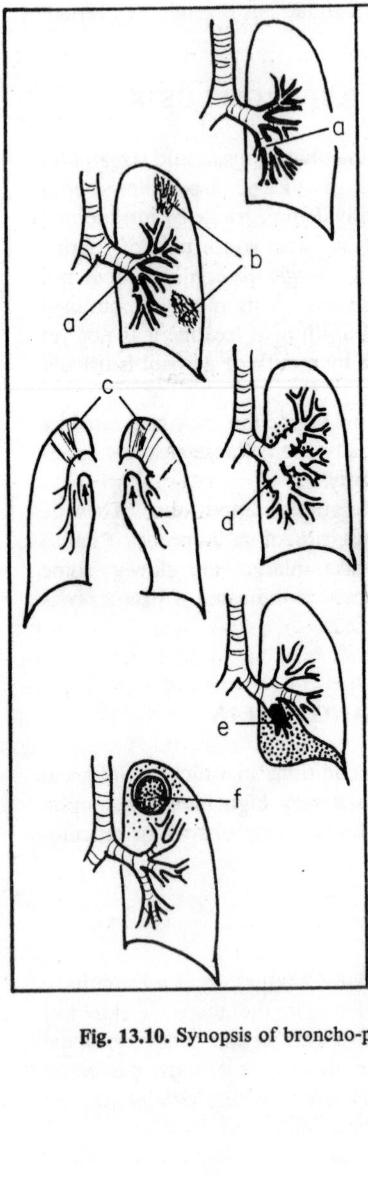

	prick test	delayed	precipitins
INCIDENTAL FINDING			
ncidental isolation from sputum	–	–	–
Isolation in atopic asthma (a)	±	–	–
ALLERGIC ASPERGILLOSIS	+	±	±
Asthma (a)			
Fleeting lung shadows (b)			
Eosinophilia			
Later:			
Upper lobe fibrosis (c)			
'Proximal' bronchiectasis (d)			
MUCOID IMPACTION			
Recurrent segmental or lobar collapse associated with aspergillus plugs and bronchial damage (e)	+	±	±
MYCETOMA (f)			
Fungus ball in cavity – from old TB, cystic disease or ? spontaneous	±	±	++
Haemoptysis or symptomless			

Fig. 13.10. Synopsis of broncho-pulmonary aspergillosis.

2. Simple pulmonary eosinophilia (Löffler's syndrome)

This term refers to a transient pulmonary reaction with reticular or nodular shadowing on the chest X-ray which may be produced by drugs (e.g. sulphonamides), and various intestinal parasites. The pulmonary changes very rarely last more than 3 or 4 weeks.

3. Tropical eosinophilia

Pulmonary eosinophilia occurring in the tropics, with or without asthma, is usually related to sensitivity to intestinal and other parasites. Filarial infestation is probably the principal cause and most cases respond to treatment with diethyl carbamazine or organic arsenicals.

4. Polyarteritis nodosa

Pulmonary eosinophilia with or without asthma may be a feature of polyarteritis nodosa. This is rare. The diagnosis will be suggested by features such as weight loss, skin rashes, peripheral neuropathy, nephritis etc.

EXTRINSIC ALLERGIC ALVEOLITIS

This term refers to hypersensitivity reactions affecting the lung parenchyma which occur in response to inhaled organic dusts. Farmer's lung is the best-known example. Usually the exposure is heavy and occupational. The reaction is an expression of Type III hypersensitivity and precipitins can generally be demonstrated in the serum. Some examples of extrinsic alveolitis are listed in Table 13.1.

TABLE 13.1. *Some examples of extrinsic allergic alveolitis*

Name	Antigen responsible
Farmer's lung	Spores of thermophyllic actinomycetes in mouldy hay.
Bird fancier's lung	Avian antigens from dust from feathers, excreta etc.
Pituitary snuff taker's lung	Porcine or bovine antigens associated with extracts of posterior pituitary.
Mushroom worker's lung	Spores of thermophyllic actinomycetes.
Maltworker's lung	Spores of *Aspergillus clavatus*.
Lung disease of grain-handlers	Dust derived from the grain weevil *Sitophilus granarius*.

Pathological features

The alveolar walls become thickened and infiltrated by lymphocytes, plasma cells and polymorphs. Small airways may show similar infiltrations. Advanced cases may show granuloma formation and variable degrees of diffuse lung fibrosis.

Clinical features

The patient may notice immediate tightness in the chest with cough and sometimes wheezing on exposure to the dust concerned. This may be mild and transient. Typically exposure is followed after an interval of about 4 hours by tachypnoea, tightness and cough. Often there is associated muscular aching, malaise, headache and fever. The relationship of the illness to the dust exposure is often not appreciated, particularly when the initial reaction is trivial and the general symptoms are pronounced. Soon after exposure there may be fine rhonchi audible on auscultation but the most constant sign in all stages is the presence of persistent fine crepitations. In advanced cases there may be constant dyspnoea and exercise limitation accompanied by cyanosis and clubbing and the picture resembles that of cryptogenic fibrosing alveolitis.

Physiological changes

A pronounced restrictive defect of ventilation is the most usual finding. Variable degrees of airways obstruction may accompany this. There may be hyperventilation and arterial hypoxaemia. Transfer factor is usually significantly reduced.

Radiological features

In early cases there may be no abnormality. During regular exposure fluffy or nodular shadowing may be seen. In advanced cases there may be areas of honeycomb change and condensed masses of granuloma and fibrous tissue which may be particularly evident in the upper lobes.

Diagnosis

The diagnosis is made from the association of the total clinical picture with exposure to a suitable organic dust. Identification of serum precipitins specific to the organic material may provide supportive evidence but results need to be interpreted with caution. In the case of Farmer's lung it should be noted that about 20 per cent of unaffected workers handling hay have serum precipitins to the thermophylic moulds responsible for the disease.

Management

Avoidance of the responsible antigen is the most important measure. This may mean a change of job or control of the exposure. It is not sufficient to advise the use of masks as these are unlikely to be used consistently by unsupervised workers. In the case of Farmer's lung improved methods of harvesting aimed at reducing the moisture content of hay are of importance. Sufferers are eligible for compensation under the Industrial Injuries Acts. Steroid therapy may be indicated on first diagnosis in a florid case but such treatment must not be viewed as an alternative to control of exposure. Little benefit can be expected in cases with advanced fibrosis.

CHAPTER 14 · DIFFUSE LUNG FIBROSIS

CRYPTOGENIC FIBROSING ALVEOLITIS
also known as Diffuse Interstitial Pulmonary Fibrosis and Hamman-Rich Syndrome

This is a rather uncommon condition in which the lung parenchyma becomes involved in a diffuse fibrotic process causing progressive impairment of gas transfer and progressive dyspnoea. The cause of the condition is not clear. It is a disease of adult life being most common in late middle age.

Pathological features

The principal features are:
1 Thickening of the alveolar walls with a tendency to increasing fibrosis.
2 'Desquamation' of large numbers of cells into the alveoli. These include macrophages and other mononuclear cells some of which may be altered Type II pneumocytes.

These changes may be irregularly dispersed within the lung and some individuals may show predominantly one form of change. As fibrosis progresses alveolar tissue becomes absorbed within condensing cellular fibrous tissue and in large parts of the lungs no alveoli may be visible at all. Because the process tends to be widespread complete collapse of large parts of lung is not generally seen; instead the lung remains aerated but the air-spaces are mainly made up of dilated bronchioles and the appearance is termed 'honeycomb lung' (Fig. 14.1).

Symptoms

In the earlier stages the patient presents with an easy panting dyspnoea and symptoms of exhaustion on effort. Sometimes an irritating unproductive cough is a prominent symptom. With progress of the disease dyspnoea can become frightening even on trivial exertion. Additional symptoms may develop due to hypoxia, cardiac failure and bronchopulmonary infection and terminally features of respiratory failure and pulmonary embolism may be added to the clinical picture.

Signs

The patient is easily dyspnoeic and may be cyanosed. Clubbing of some degree is seen in about two-thirds of cases. The most consistent finding is the presence of fine crepitations on auscultation of the chest. These tend to occur throughout inspiration being especially marked towards the end of inspiration.

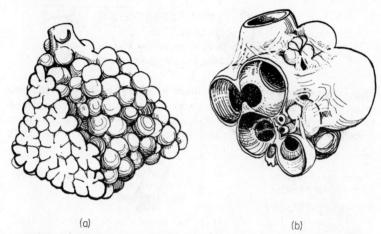

(a)   (b)

Fig. 14.1. *Honeycomb lung.* A three-dimensional impression of the structure of the normal lobule (a) and of the air spaces in advanced lung fibrosis (honeycomb lung) (b). There is dense fibrosis with disappearance of normal lung architecture. The air spaces are thick walled and much larger than alveoli. Most of them probably represent dilated terminal and respiratory bronchioles.

Physiological changes

1. SPIROMETRY
A restrictive ventilatory defect is almost always evident by the time troublesome symptoms are reported.

2. LUNG VOLUMES
All lung volumes are reduced but tend to maintain their relative proportions.

3. LUNG COMPLIANCE
This is reduced. Measurement is not essential to the diagnosis.

4. BLOOD GASES

At rest blood gases tend to be normal until the disease is well advanced when arterial hypoxaemia and hypocapnia (low Pco_2 due to hyperventilation) are generally found. Exercise is limited by arterial hypoxaemia and exercise tolerance may be extended by breathing oxygen-enriched air.

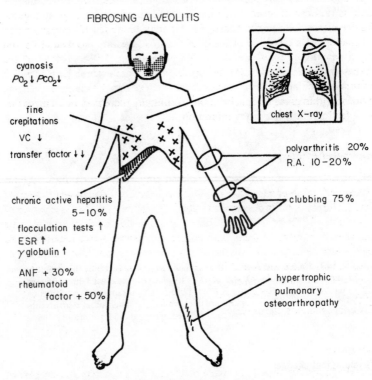

Fig. 14.2. *Summary of features of fibrosing alveolitis.*

5. GAS TRANSFER

There is characteristically a pronounced impairment of transfer factor (p. 61). It is common to find values of around 5 ml/min/mmHg (normal values above 20 ml/min/mmHg depending on age and stature). Traditionally the defective gas transfer has been regarded as a 'diffusion defect' due to thickening of the alveolar membrane. This explanation is undoubtedly an oversimplification and it seems likely that other mechanisms are more important and these include:

a A much extended range of ventilation/perfusion ratios throughout the lungs due to irregularly distributed stiffness (p. 19).

b Replacement of alveoli by fibrous tissue resulting in overall reduction in alveolar surface and capillary blood volume.

Radiological changes

The appearances vary somewhat depending upon the stage of the disease and its rapidity of onset. The most usual features are (1) a 'ground-glass' haziness especially at the bases. To this may be added (2) streaky wisps of shadow with elevation of the diaphragms suggesting basal collapse and (3) a generalised micronodular (miliary) mottling. The end-stage of the disease is characterised by (4) the appearances of 'honeycomb lung' in which multiple circular areas of translucency 2 to 5 mm in diameter become evident within areas of opacification. Terminally there may be changes due to infection and pulmonary infarction.

Associated disorders

The E.S.R. is usually elevated. Associated polyarthritis is common. About 10 per cent of cases may have rheumatoid arthritis and a positive rheumatoid factor is found in the serum in about 50 per cent of cases. Elevation of γ-globulins is fairly frequently found and the flocculation tests may be positive. A number of cases with coexisting chronic active hepatitis have been described. Antinuclear factor may be present and other non-organ specific antibodies are found in about 30 per cent of cases. A higher than expected incidence of thyroid disease has been reported. The relationship between cryptogenic fibrosing alveolitis and other collagen or autoimmune disorders remains conjectural.

Diagnosis

The diagnosis can usually be made on clinical grounds with the support of radiological appearances and simple tests of pulmonary function including measurement of transfer factor.

In a typical patient the diagnosis may be straightforward: a middle-aged individual with progressive panting dyspnoea and cyanosis but with no evidence of cardiac disease or airways obstruction is found to have clubbing and diffuse crepitations and a reticulo-nodular pattern of shadowing on the chest X-ray which is more pronounced at the bases; spirometry reveals a much restricted vital capacity but good early-expiratory flow rate and transfer factor is found to be markedly impaired.

DIFFERENTIAL DIAGNOSIS
In less typical cases the differential diagnosis is potentially lengthy.

Miliary mottling is discussed on p. 69. Some of the more important alternatives are:

1. *Extrinsic allergic alveolitis* (p. 137). It is very important to differentiate this preventable form of alveolitis. Clinical, radiological and physiological features may be identical; points of difference are: (a) history of exposure to appropriate organic dust and presence of serum precipitins; (b) more prominent involvement of upper lobes in extrinsic alveolitis; (c) rheumatoid factor, ANF and elevation of γ-globulin are commonly found in cryptogenic fibrosing alveolitis.

2. *Bronchiectasis*. Basal crepitations, clubbing and irregular basal shadowing on the chest X-ray may cause confusion. Points of difference are: (a) cough is longstanding and productive of large amounts of purulent sputum; (b) dyspnoea if present is usually a consequence of airways obstruction; (c) cyanosis is uncommon and generally associated with chronic ventilatory failure; (d) transfer factor is not usually reduced.

3. *Chronic left heart failure*. May rarely produce reticulo-nodular shadowing and dyspnoea; clinical, radiological and ECG changes of left heart disease will generally be present.

4. *Sarcoidosis*. Differentiation may be difficult without a positive Kveim test or other features of sarcoidosis particularly in the skin and eye (p. 153). In diffuse sarcoidosis of the lungs the defect in transfer factor is often more modest than would be expected from the radiographic changes.

5. *Lymphangitis carcinomatosa*. This may produce progressive dyspnoea with striking impairment of transfer factor. There will usually be past or present evidence of carcinoma—usually an adenocarcinoma.

6. *Pulmonary embolism*. This should rarely cause confusion but repeated embolism should always be borne in mind in any patient with progressive obscure breathlessness and basal shadowing on the chest X-ray.

LUNG BIOPSY
Biopsy confirmation of the diagnosis is not essential when the diagnosis or a particular line of action is clear. Sometimes however a therapeutic decision is impossible without a histological diagnosis.

Open-lung biopsy
This allows removal of a relatively large specimen which can be selected from a moderately affected part of the lung. The disadvantages are the hazards of anaesthetic, thoracotomy and subsequent convalescence.

Closed-lung biopsy
A number of needle techniques have been developed for obtaining specimens of aerated lung. The Jack needle shears off a tiny fragment of lung snagged by small hooks on the stylet. Steel's lung trephine is operated by a high-speed air drill and cuts a small core of lung tissue. In most instances the

disturbance is slight; only about a third of patients develop a pneumo-thorax and of these less than half require pleural intubation. Trans-bronchial biopsy performed by fine biopsy forceps passed through a fibre-optic bronchoscope and wedged in a peripheral bronchiole offers an alternative relatively safe means of obtaining multiple samples of lung parenchyma in the diagnosis of diffuse lung disease. The main drawbacks of closed biopsy are the small size of the specimen and occasional failure to obtain a specimen.

Course of the disease

The course is very variable. A small number of patients have a rapidly progressive course over only a few months and the illness may be accom-panied by severe malaise and pneumonic features. A slower downhill course is more usual over a period of years. In some elderly individuals the condition is discovered by chance and appears to be completely stationary.

Treatment

CORTICOSTEROID TREATMENT

Patients with disturbing dyspnoea or clear evidence of progression should be treated with corticosteroids. It is usual to use a large dose (40 to 60 mg daily) for a period of up to 3 months if the disease threatens to disable. If any improvement is to be achieved it will generally be evident by this time. The dose is then progressively reduced to the lowest level capable of maintaining the improvement.

RESULTS

Improvement of some degree is seen in about two-thirds of cases receiving corticosteroid treatment. The more acute the mode of onset and the youn-ger the patient, the more likely it is that there will be a worthwhile improve-ment. However a worthwhile response may be seen even in advanced disease with honeycomb change.

IMMUNOSUPPRESSIVE THERAPY

Azathioprine may have some effect on the disease and may be useful where there are especially compelling reasons for avoiding large doses of prednisone.

OXYGEN

This may be useful in advanced disease when even gentle exercise is poorly tolerated. A stationary cylinder in the house and long lengths of plastic piping may enable the patient to negotiate the stairs or take a bath which might otherwise be impossible. A rechargeable portable cylinder may extend the range of activities out of doors.

SUPPORTIVE MEASURES

Measures to control infection, heart failure and exhausting cough are required as the disease progresses. Opiates may be necessary to control terrifying terminal dyspnoea.

DIFFUSE FIBROSIS DUE TO DRUGS AND POISONS

Busulphan

Diffuse pneumonitis may rarely occur during the treatment of chronic myeloid leukaemia with this drug—often after many months of treatment. Diffuse fibrosis may follow but sometimes withdrawal of the drug results in resolution of the reaction with or without corticosteroid treatment.

Bleomycin

An acute pulmonary reaction resembling pulmonary oedema may complicate treatment with this cytostatic antibiotic used in cancer chemotherapy and the reaction may be followed by diffuse pulmonary fibrosis.

Nitrofurantoin

Two types of parenchymal lung reaction are encountered in association with this drug, one acute and one insidious in onset. The second variety is characterised by widespread diffuse pulmonary fibrosis.

Methysergide

This drug (used in the treatment of severe migraine) may produce pleural fibrosis which may be nodular and which may involve the lung to a variable degree.

Paraquat

Poisoning with the weedkiller paraquat induces a vicious accelerated form of diffuse lung fibrosis in which the whole range of fibrosing alveolitis, from the earliest changes to widespread honeycombing, may be condensed into a period of less than three weeks by which time death from hypoxia has usually supervened. Very occasionally individuals may escape with lung changes arrested at an intermediate stage. Fatal poisoning follows accidental consumption of only a mouthful of agricultural concentrate (Gramoxone). Accidental poisoning with diluted material or the more generally available paraquat/diquat mixture in granular form is almost unheard of. Intentional self-poisoning with various preparations accounts for about half of the fatalities.

Radiation

Therapeutic irradiation which involves the lung fields may lead to an acute pneumonitis which generally resolves within a few weeks. A variable degree of fibrosis may follow over subsequent months in the distribution of the irradiated areas.

Occupational causes (see p. 215)

RHEUMATOID ARTHRITIS

The pulmonary accompaniments of rheumatoid arthritis are summarised in Fig. 14.3.

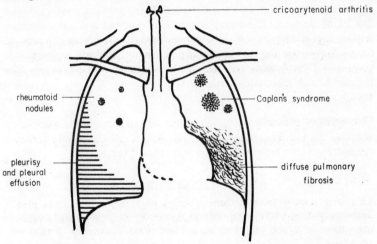

Fig. 14.3. *Summary of pulmonary complications of rheumatoid arthritis.*

Pleurisy and pleural effusion

These are common in rheumatoid arthritis and may tend to be recurrent. Effusions are rarely large.

Pulmonary fibrosis

This is much less common, probably occurring in no more than 2 per cent of cases. There is a definite but ill-understood relationship between rheumatoid arthritis and fibrosing alveolitis. The fibrosis accompanying rheumatoid arthritis may appear to be stationary for many years. If pulmonary fibrosis is disabling or progressive, treatment with cortico-steroids may be indicated.

Pulmonary nodules

These are not common. The appearance is of several soft spherical nodules up to 1 cm in diameter and this may lead to the erroneous diagnosis of metastatic malignant disease. The nodules have the same histology as rheumatoid nodules elsewhere; they sometimes cavitate and may disappear spontaneously.

Caplan's syndrome

Rheumatoid arthritis occurring in association with coalworkers' pneumoconiosis may be marked by the occurrence of very large pulmonary nodules 2–3 cm in diameter. These may also break down and cavitate sometimes leading to the suspicion of tuberculosis though tubercle bacilli are not found. Sometimes the rheumatoid arthritis is not clinically evident until years later. Other pneumoconioses may be associated with massive nodules in patients with rheumatoid arthritis.

Cricoarytenoid arthritis

This may lead to hoarseness or occasionally inspiratory stridor.

SYSTEMIC SCLEROSIS

This uncommon condition produces a number of pulmonary complications most of which only become evident when the disease is relatively advanced.

Diffuse pulmonary fibrosis

The clinical, radiological and physiological features of this are like those of fibrosing alveolitis although there is some evidence that the alteration of fibrous tissue may be of a fundamentally different nature in systemic sclerosis.

Restriction of chest wall movement

This late complication may arise as a consequence of severe thickening and contraction of the skin of the trunk.

Inhalation pneumonia

Pneumonia and lung abscess may result from overspill from a dilated oesophagus secondary to stricture formation. Pneumonia is a common terminal event.

The diagnosis is made by recognition of the characteristic changes in the skin and other organs. Where pulmonary fibrosis appears to be causing disability, corticosteroid treatment is generally tried—almost always with disappointing results.

SYSTEMIC LUPUS ERYTHEMATOSUS (SLE)

The pulmonary complications of this uncommon multi-system disorder are as follows:

Pleurisy

Pleurisy, sometimes with a small effusion, is common and may be the presenting feature. Pleurisy occurring in young female patients who are more ill than might be expected and who have a high E.S.R. should lead to suspicion of SLE.

Pneumonia

Patchy recurrent pneumonia is a common feature of SLE in relapse. Usually the patient is ill and there may be a characteristic rash, arthritis and other features of the disease. The diagnosis will be supported by the finding of antinuclear factor, LE cells and DNA antibody in the serum.

'Small lung syndrome'

It is uncertain whether true diffuse pulmonary fibrosis occurs in association with SLE but patients may complain of dyspnoea associated with a sensation of restriction within the chest. There may be no definite physical signs or radiological features but spirometry may reveal a restrictive ventilatory defect and transfer factor may be moderately impaired. The syndrome tends to resolve fairly promptly with steroid treatment.

CHAPTER 15 · SARCOIDOSIS

The definition of sarcoidosis is based upon the presence of granulomatous tissue with a characteristic histological picture found in characteristic areas of the body. The diagnosis rests upon identification of clinical features and in practice histological confirmation is not always necessary.

The histological picture

The characteristic cell is a largish epithelioid cell with a pale staining nucleus arranged in clumps or whorls of varying size and bounded by a sparse zone of lymphocytic infiltration. The clumps of typical cells all look strikingly the same in the various affected tissues. Caseation is not seen even in the centre of quite large masses; but hyaline degeneration may merge with areas of fibrosis. Occasional giant cells are present and some may be seen to contain concentric inclusion bodies (Schaumann bodies).

Aetiology

The aetiology is not known. It is no longer regarded as a neoplastic type of reticuloendothelial proliferation akin to Hodgkin's disease and discussion centres on the possibility that it represents an atypical response to the tubercle bacillus (and possibly other agents which are capable of producing granulomata) or that it may be due to an unidentified transmissible agent.

A striking feature of cases of sarcoidosis is evidence of defective cellularly mediated (Type IV) hypersensitivity. It may be difficult or impossible to induce a response to tuberculin or other agents normally capable of evoking this response. The production of humoral antibody by lymphocytes is unimpaired. Exposure to beryllium has in the past produced granulomata indistinguishable from those of sarcoidosis (exposure is now very strictly controlled).

Clinical manifestations

It is useful to consider the clinical manifestations under two headings:
1 Acute manifestations in the young which are generally benign and

characterised by bilateral hilar lymph node enlargement (BHL) and erythema nodosum.

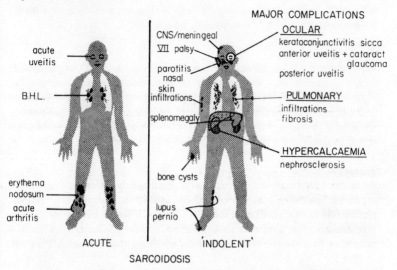

Fig. 15.1. *Summary of the principal clinical features of sarcoidosis.*

2   Chronic or recurrent manifestations, which tend to occur in an older age-group, involve many tissues of the body and include infiltration and fibrosis of the lungs.

BHL AND ERYTHEMA NODOSUM

This is by far the commonest manifestation of sarcoidosis. Sarcoidosis is the commonest cause of erythema nodosum in young adults. Sometimes general malaise, mild fever and arthralgia precede the erythema nodosum for a week or two. Other accompaniments of this acute form of sarcoidosis are acute arthritis of ankles, knees or wrists with marked oedema and reddening, parotid enlargement and acute anterior uveitis. There are no signs on examination of the chest and there is no disturbance of pulmonary function.

Diagnosis

BHL accompanied by erythema nodosum is always due to sarcoidosis and no further investigations are really necessary. Where BHL is found without any helpful clues there is still rarely real difficulty in diagnosis. If BHL is slight there may be difficulty in distinguishing the appearances from those of unusually prominent pulmonary arteries. Hodgkin's disease is sometimes suspected but this almost never shows the striking symmetry of the

BHL of sarcoidosis and it is exceedingly rare for hilar adenopathy to be the sole manifestation of Hodgkin's disease. In cases of serious doubt tuberculin and Kveim tests may be helpful (but not infallible) and lymph node biopsy or mediastinoscopy may be necessary.

Course
The prognosis is excellent. Erythema nodosum and arthralgia subside within a month and uveitis rarely persists much longer. Radiological signs of BHL may persist for 2 or 3 years but generally resolve over about 18 months. Occasionally some flecks of pulmonary infiltrate are seen to come and go during this time but only a very small percentage of cases go on to develop the more indolent forms of sarcoidosis.

Treatment
As a rule no treatment is necessary. Particularly severe arthralgia or erythema nodosum may be helped by aspirin or butazolidine or even prednisone in modest dosage for 2 to 3 weeks. There is usually no call for hospitalisation or intensive follow up both of which foster concern and neurosis which may be potentially more disabling than the condition itself.

PULMONARY INFILTRATIONS IN SARCOIDOSIS
Limited infiltrations may appear in the course of evolution of BHL with erythema nodosum but major involvement of the lungs in sarcoidosis tends to be encountered when there is already evidence of indolent sarcoidosis in various tissues of the body (see Fig. 15.1). Not all chronic indolent sarcoidosis passes through an acute phase with BHL and erythema nodosum—indeed this evolution may be rare.

Radiological appearances
These are of mottling often affecting the mid-zones principally and the mottling may be formed in radially-arranged leashes. In some instances there is generalised finer stippling.

Physiological changes
A modest restrictive defect and some reduction in transfer factor is usual if changes are widespread but the defect often seems slight when compared with the X-ray appearances (cf. Fibrosing alveolitis, p. 141).

PULMONARY FIBROSIS
This is quite rare. It usually involves the mid-zones most severely. The X-ray appearances are of contraction of lung volume and fine spider's web-like linear shadows with areas of condensed shadowing which may contain honeycomb spaces or larger cysts. Physiological tests reflect the changes; lung volumes are small, there is a severe restrictive ventilatory defect and

serious impairment of transfer factor. Exercise is limited and there may be cyanosis. Clubbing is a rarity.

Course of parenchymal changes
Infiltrations often remain stationary for years. Perhaps a quarter of patients with extensive infiltration develop some fibrosis which may also remain constant for long periods and may not be associated with severe symptoms. Probably less than 10 per cent with such infiltrations become disabled and a smaller proportion actually die from pulmonary involvement.

EXTRAPULMONARY SARCOIDOSIS
Some of the commoner sites are indicated diagrammatically in Fig. 15.1 and a few deserve special mention.

Ocular sarcoidosis
Anterior uveitis (iridocyclitis) is the commonest manifestation. It may be obvious because of pain, misting vision and the presence of ciliary injection but sometimes it is only revealed by slit-lamp inspection. Posterior uveitis (perivenous sheathing and chorioretinitis) is much less common. Uveitis occurs in about a quarter of all patients with sarcoidosis and sarcoidosis accounts for about 5 per cent of uveitis presenting to ophthalmologists. Keratoconjunctivitis sicca and lacrimal gland enlargement may complicate chronic sarcoidosis.

Uveoparotid fever
This is the name given to a syndrome of uveitis, parotid gland enlargement and sometimes facial nerve palsy (usually temporary).

Central nervous system involvement
Facial palsy may also be due to meningeal involvement which may produce a variety of obscure neurological syndromes and epilepsy.

Skin involvement
Lupus pernio is a chilblain-like lesion occurring in violaceous patches on the face and limbs and it is generally accompanied by pulmonary involvement. Nodules of sarcoid granuloma may occur in the skin particularly in old scars.

Bone involvement
Bone cysts are the hallmark of established indolent sarcoidosis. Digits are commonly involved. If affected, the digit is swollen; there is no point in routinely X-raying the hands in suspected sarcoidosis.

Calcium metabolism

Chronic sarcoidosis may disturb calcium metabolism and lead to hypercalcaemia, hypercalcuria, renal stones and even nephrocalcinosis.

Diagnosis

Where a number of features occur together the diagnosis may be straightforward. Where lung involvement appears to be solitary, biopsy of the lung, liver or lymph nodes may be justified.

TUBERCULIN TESTS (p. 92)

There are negative results in over three-quarters of all patients with sarcoidosis.

KVEIM TEST

An intradermal injection of a suspension of an extract of human sarcoid spleen is made into the skin and the site marked (e.g. by tattooing). After 6 weeks the site is inspected and biopsied. A positive result is indicated by the presence of sarcoid granuloma. Individual extracts have differing records of reliability but generally over three-quarters of patients give positive results. 'False positive' results may be found in Crohn's disease and a number of disorders associated with enlargement of lymph nodes.

Treatment

The great majority of patients with sarcoidosis require no treatment at all.

The generally accepted indications for treatment with oral steroids are:

1. SEVERE UVEITIS

Where uveitis cannot be adequately controlled by topical steroid treatment oral prednisone may be necessary and this is the commonest indication for such treatment.

2. PROGRESSIVE PULMONARY CHANGES

Where there is clinical, radiological and physiological evidence of deterioration it is usual to start treatment with oral steroids. X-ray signs of infiltration often resolve promptly with little change in physiological function but sometimes with improvement in dyspnoea and cough. There is no convincing evidence that protracted control of radiological infiltrations with steroid treatment averts development of fibrosis.

3. HYPERCALCAEMIA

Carries the threat of ultimate renal failure and it is usually controlled by a modest dose of oral steroid.

Skin manifestations of sarcoidosis may be amenable to local treatment by steroid creams or infiltration which is worthwhile in cosmetically strategic areas.

4. IMPORTANT NEUROLOGICAL INVOLVEMENT

CHAPTER 16 · CHRONIC BRONCHITIS, AIRWAYS OBSTRUCTION AND EMPHYSEMA

Definitions

CHRONIC BRONCHITIS. Chronic cough with production of sputum on most days for at least 3 months in the year for at least 2 years

The term refers simply to the symptoms of cough and sputum (generally excluding that due to some localised lesion in the lungs). Simple chronic bronchitis is not accompanied by shortness of breath.

AIRWAYS OBSTRUCTION. Diffuse airways narrowing causing increased resistance to airflow

The expression denotes a disturbance of physiology and airways obstruction is generally confirmed by physiological tests. Airways obstruction commonly accompanies chronic bronchitis and is generally responsible for the dyspnoea. Airways obstruction in chronic bronchitis is *not* necessarily due to emphysema.

EMPHYSEMA. Dilatation of the terminal air-spaces of the lungs distal to the terminal bronchiole with destruction of their walls

The term denotes a pathological lesion, not a clinical syndrome. Dyspnoea which occurs in association with chronic bronchitis is *not* necessarily due to emphysema. It is generally not possible to diagnose the presence of emphysema reliably in life on clinical grounds alone. Generalised emphysema is always accompanied by evidence of airways obstruction.

ASTHMA. A disease characterised by variable dyspnoea due to widespread narrowing of the peripheral airways in the lungs, varying in severity over short periods of time, either spontaneously or as a result of treatment

As some patients with asthma present with chronic cough productive of sputum and as airways obstruction is a principal feature, it is to be expected that some patients with asthma may unintentionally be included in the group of diseases discussed here (see p. 165).

CHRONIC OBSTRUCTIVE LUNG DISEASE (C.O.L.D.)

This term, and others rather like it, have grown into common use as a means of indicating the common clinical situation in which all of the above phenomena may be inextricably mixed. The term is convenient but lacks precision and fosters the misconception that there is a single uniform disease entity in which all elements are necessarily present. Where it appears in this chapter it should be taken to mean 'chronic bronchitis accompanied by diffuse airways obstruction with or without emphysema'.

Prevalence

1 In the United Kingdom chronic bronchitis as defined occurs in about 8 per cent of men and 3 per cent of women. The ratio of males to females increases with age.
2 A huge amount of loss of work is attributable to chronic bronchitis (about 36 million working days each year).
3 The prevalence is much higher in the United Kingdom than in other countries.

Mortality

1 In the United Kingdom more than 30,000 persons die from C.O.L.D. each year.
2 Mortality rises steeply with age but more than 8,500 of the deaths occur before retirement age.
3 The mortality from C.O.L.D. is much higher than in other countries.

Aetiology

It is not possible to identify a single cause of chronic bronchitis and its accompaniments but a number of factors are known to be involved.

CIGARETTE SMOKING
Cigarette smoking is of major importance in the genesis of chronic bronchitis.

1. *Symptoms*
Symptoms of simple bronchitis in the general population are:
a common in smokers

b related to the number of cigarettes smoked per day
c exceptional in non-smokers.

2. Simple ventilatory tests
Smokers, as a group, have lower performance than non-smokers of comparable age; the severity of the impairment being proportional to the number of cigarettes smoked per day.

3. Morbidity
Work-loss and hospital admissions are much more frequent in smokers and related to the number of cigarettes smoked per day.

4. Mortality
The mortality from C.O.L.D. is much higher amongst smokers. The risk of death from C.O.L.D. in a man smoking 15 cigarettes daily is 12 times that of a non-smoker. In a man smoking 30 cigarettes daily the risk is 20 times that of a non-smoker.

ATMOSPHERIC POLLUTION

Long-term
1 Prevalence of symptoms, morbidity and mortality from C.O.L.D. are related to the degree of urbanisation. They are also related to mean levels of atmospheric pollution which seems likely to be the most important element within urbanisation in this context.
2 In non-smokers the effect of urbanisation and atmospheric pollution is very small.
3 In smokers the adverse effects of atmospheric pollution become increasingly marked in proportion to smoking exposure which suggests an interaction between these factors.

Short-term
Exceptional episodes of heavy pollution have been associated with greatly increased numbers of admissions to hospitals and deaths because of C.O.L.D.

SOCIO-ECONOMIC FACTORS
Mortality from C.O.L.D. as judged from death certification is inversely related to socio-economic status. Mortality in the Registrar General's Class V is six times greater than in Class II.

INFECTION
Virus infections are known to be associated with some exacerbations of C.O.L.D. and bacterial infection of the sputum is a feature of established

exacerbations. These infections may play an important role in the progress of the disease but there is no good evidence to support a causative role.

CONSTITUTIONAL FACTORS

Familial tendencies to C.O.L.D. are sometimes encountered but the effects of shared smoking habits, atmospheric pollution and social class obscure the relationship. Unrecognised asthma may sometimes underlie the familial tendency.

A very rare form of emphysema is due to an inherited deficiency of α-1-antitrypsin, a component of normal plasma globulin.

REGIONAL FACTORS

Chronic bronchitis and its accompaniments is very much more common in the U.K. than in most other countries. The reasons for this are probably complex and include the effect of differing diagnostic conventions.

Within the U.K. the prevalence and mortality from C.O.L.D. tends to be higher in the North and West compared with the South and East even when allowance is made for the effects of urbanisation.

Clinical features and progress of the disease

SIMPLE CHRONIC BRONCHITIS

The progress of simple bronchitis is generally insidious. Cough which may be present initially only during the first part of the day in winter months may, over several years, come to last all day throughout the year. Occasional patients relate the onset of symptoms to a single severe respiratory tract infection.

ACUTE EXACERBATIONS

Particularly in relation to colds, patients with chronic bronchitis develop increased cough productive of yellow purulent sputum with mild symptoms of general malaise. The illness may last a few days or several weeks.

DEVELOPMENT OF AIRWAYS OBSTRUCTION

Not all patients with simple chronic bronchitis develop airways obstruction. The cardinal symptom is dyspnoea which may be accompanied by wheezing and is generally related to effort. Dyspnoea is commonly noted for the first time after an acute exacerbation. Clinical and spirometric evidence of airways obstruction is common in patients who are quite unaware of any symptom apart from cough. Airways obstruction is often already severe when medical attention is sought for the first time.

SYMPTOMS OF BRONCHIAL HYPERREACTIVITY

Bronchial hyperreactivity produces symptoms associated with airways obstruction and may help to distinguish dyspnoea due to this cause. The patient complains of sensations of tightness, choking or paroxysms of coughing when confronted by smoke, cold air, fog, car exhaust and other fumes. Symptoms are often related to particular weather conditions.

PROGRESS OF DISABILITY

There is generally a very gradual progression of disability extending over 10 to 40 years. It may become apparent through increasing absence from work, gradual limitation of exercise tolerance and a reduced range of activities (p. 32). The prognosis is related to severity of exercise limitation; 40 per cent of patients who are required to walk at a reduced pace on flat ground die within 5 years.

With time, acute exacerbations become more alarming and are accompanied by breathlessness at rest, and difficulty in expectoration; admission to hospital may be required during these episodes.

CLINICAL PATTERNS IN SEVERE CHRONIC
OBSTRUCTIVE LUNG DISEASE

Two patterns of disturbance may be discerned during the progress of advanced C.O.L.D. which differ mainly in the extent to which ventilatory drive is preserved in the face of increasing airways obstruction. The main features are summarised in Figs. 16.1 and 16.2. Most patients do not fit either pattern completely but have some features of both.

Type A ('pink puffer')

In this group ventilatory drive is well preserved even in the presence of very severe airways obstruction. Dyspnoea may be intense. Blood gases are maintained in the normal range at rest until terminally.

Type B ('blue bloater')

Individuals meeting this description have poor respiratory drive and easily drift into respiratory failure with elevation of $P\mathrm{co_2}$, hypoxia and heart failure particularly during infective exacerbations.

In simple terms the 'pink puffer' can be regarded as 'doing his best' to breathe enough to keep the $P\mathrm{co_2}$ down often in the face of great difficulties whilst the 'blue bloater' 'gives up' at a relatively early stage and settles for poor blood gases when he could breathe more 'if he tried harder'.

The reasons for the early ventilatory failure of Type B patients are not clear.

Emphysema

1 The term emphysema (defined p. 156) refers to a form of parenchymal lung damage and not to a clinical syndrome.
2 It is difficult to diagnose reliably.
3 Whether or not a patient has emphysema is not clinically very important—the management of the patient will only exceptionally be affected by the diagnosis.
4 Emphysema is widely over-diagnosed on inadequate evidence.
5 As emphysema is untreatable the diagnosis tends to foster an air of hopelessness in the management.

Pathological features

Two principal patterns are seen (Fig. 16.3, p. 165).

1. CENTRILOBULAR OR CENTRIACINAR EMPHYSEMA

Here the distension and damage affect the respiratory bronchioles; the more distal alveolar ducts and alveoli tend to be well preserved.

2. PANACINAR EMPHYSEMA

Here the distension and destruction appear to involve the whole of the acinus.

3. IRREGULAR EMPHYSEMA

This term is used to describe the very common appearance of scarring and damage which affect the parenchyma patchily without particular regard for acinar structure.

CLINICO-PATHOLOGICAL RELATIONSHIPS

Centrilobular emphysema of modest extent is very common and not necessarily associated with disability. More severe degrees are associated with prominent bronchitic symptoms, disturbance of ventilation—perfusion relationships and hypoxia. This may be due to the relatively well-preserved blood supply to the badly ventilated alveoli beyond the damaged zone.

Severe panacinar emphysema is less common. The elastic network of the normal lung is badly disorganised, the lung becomes floppy leading to a severe degree of airways obstruction particularly during expiration. Changes in the blood gases tend to be less drastic perhaps because the blood supply in damaged areas is reduced in proportion to the reduced ventilation to these areas. Ventilatory drive is generally better preserved than in cases with severe centrilobular emphysema. It is tempting to associate the 'pink puffer' with panacinar emphysema and the 'blue bloater' with centrilobular emphysema; available evidence suggests that

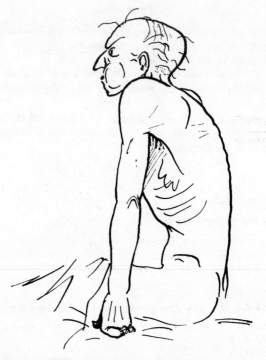

Fig. 16.1. *Type A or 'Pink puffer'—the picture of good respiratory drive.*

Individuals in this category tend to have the following features:
    Intense dyspnoea often with purse-lip breathing
    Thin and often elderly
    Small sputum volume
    Rarely develop oedema or overt heart failure.
Investigation may show:
    Near-normal blood gas values (until terminally)
    Very severe airways obstruction
    Increased total lung capacity
    Radiological evidence of emphysema
    Impairment of transfer factor.

this is an oversimplification but that some sort of loose relationship may exist.

Which patients have emphysema?

CENTRILOBULAR EMPHYSEMA

There are no helpful clinical or radiological features which allow the

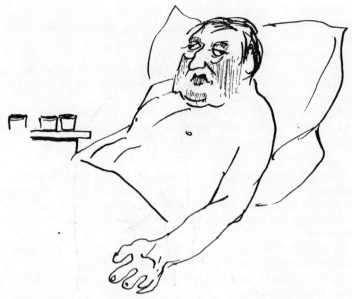

Fig. 16.2. *Type B or 'Blue bloater'—the picture of poor respiratory drive.*

Individuals in this category tend to have the following features:
    Relatively mild dyspnoea
    Often obese
    Large sputum volume and frequent infective exacerbations
    Often oedematous and easily lapse into congestive heart failure.
Investigation may show:
    Abnormal blood gases—hypercapnia, hypoxaemia with elevated plasma
        bicarbonate and polycythaemia
    Sometimes only moderately severe airways obstruction
    Fairly normal total lung capacity
    No radiological evidence of emphysema
    Little or no reduction in transfer factor.

diagnosis of centrilobular emphysema although there are clinical situations in which its presence may be suspected.

PANACINAR EMPHYSEMA

(a) Clinical

Most of the hallowed signs of emphysema are merely those of over-inflation which may accompany airways obstruction of any sort. Emphysema may be suspected when the features of Type A are encountered (Fig. 16.1).

(b) Radiological
The following features are strongly suggestive of severe panacinar emphysema.
1   Bullae evident on chest X-ray.
2   Deficiency of blood vessel markings in the peripheral half of the lung fields in most areas seen on PA chest X-ray compared with relatively easily seen more proximal vessels.

These features will often be accompanied by evidence of severe over-inflation—low flattened diaphragms on the PA film and a large retro-sternal air-space on the lateral film.

Note (a) When interpreting a reported radiological diagnosis of emphysema it is important to know the criteria used by the radiologist. Many radiologists equate the signs of mere overinflation with the presence of emphysema and such signs can be completely reversible if the patient has asthma.

(b) Radiological diagnosis of panacinar emphysema is only possible when the disease is advanced.

(c) Widespread emphysema of any type may be present despite a normal chest X-ray.

Management of chronic obstructive lung disease

1. Smoking
Patients should always be urged to stop smoking even when they insist that it helps them to produce sputum. Symptoms of simple chronic bronchitis may disappear but there is often no change in the symptoms in the case of more advanced disease. Patients should not be led to expect improvement or ensuing disappointment will be followed by resumption of the habit.

2. Detection of unsuspected asthma
A proportion of patients diagnosed as having chronic bronchitis and airways obstruction may show dramatic improvement in respiratory symptoms when treated with corticosteroids—suggesting an 'allergic' or 'asthmatic' component. It is extremely important that such individuals should not be overlooked.

Trial of steroids
Prednisone 15 mg daily for a fortnight is sufficient to determine whether

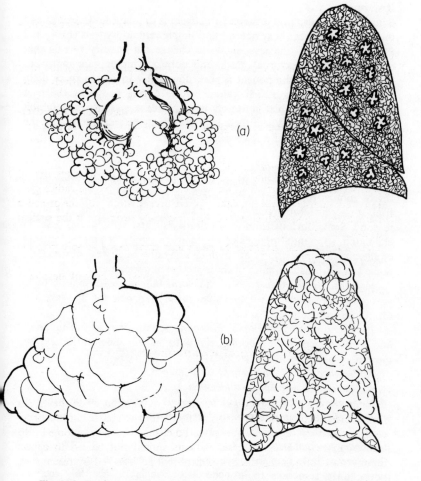

(a)

(b)

Fig. 16.3. *Emphysema.* Diagrammatic view of lobule and whole lung section in (a) centrilobular and (b) panacinar emphysema.

or not there is responsive disease. Prednisone in this dose for such a short duration is virtually devoid of harmful effects and minimal fuss should accompany the prescribing of the drugs; if there is no response then it may be stopped abruptly. A trial of steroid therapy should be carried out at a time when the patient is in a stable state rather than during recovery from an infective exacerbation.

Assessment

Sometimes the response to steroid treatment is dramatic and obvious and there is improvement in symptoms and simple ventilatory tests (FEV_1 and PEFR). Sometimes the tests show no change but enquiry reveals that exercise tolerance, nocturnal attacks and morning symptoms are improved. It is useful to give the patient a peak flow meter to record twice daily morning and evening PEFR values before, during and after the trial period. Acute bronchial infection with purulent sputum may inhibit response to steroids. Where there is doubt it may be worth repeating the trial after an interval of a few weeks.

Who requires trial of steroids?

It could be argued that all patients who have chronic airways obstruction severe enough to interfere with their daily activities merit a therapeutic trial. It may be more practical to limit such a trial to those most likely to respond. Some obvious features which may suggest asthma are: onset in childhood, substantial periods of normality, a family or personal history of allergies, a family history of anything suggestive of airways obstruction. Some less obvious attributes of those who may respond are:

1. *Relatively short duration of dyspnoea.* Individuals dyspnoeic for 5 years are more likely to respond than those dyspnoeic for 25 years (except those with very early onset).

2. *Severe morning symptoms.* The more severe symptoms of tightness and breathlessness in the morning relative to the remainder of the day, the more likely is a response to steroids.

3. *Presence of eosinophilia in blood or sputum.*

4. *Nocturnal cough and breathlessness.*

5. *Tendency to be worse in summer*—but a tendency to be worse in winter is of little help in forecasting responsiveness.

Pulmonary function tests

These are of little help in forecasting responsiveness to steroids in this group; huge responses to bronchodilator inhalation are only seen in asthma, but lesser degrees of 'reversibility' do not discriminate (pp. 120–1).

3. Antibiotic and chemotherapy

WHEN?

1   All patients with chronic bronchitis should receive treatment with a broad spectrum antibiotic during infective exacerbations—that is when the sputum is persistently purulent (yellowish or green) and increased in quantity above the usual. Antibiotic treatment shortens exacerbations and may prevent lung damage.

2 Treatment should be started promptly. It may be helpful for some patients to have a small stock of antibiotic at home so that there need be no delay in starting treatment.

3 There is no need to culture the sputum in an infective exacerbation unless the patient is gravely ill or the response to treatment is unsatisfactory. If the sputum becomes purulent it is generally safe to assume that the responsible organisms are the pneumococcus and *Haemophilus influenzae*.

4 If the sputum is mucoid in appearance there is usually no need to prescribe an antibiotic whatever the bacteriological results.

WHICH ANTIBIOTIC?

There is little to choose between the following:

Amoxycillin 250 mg three times daily *or*

Cotrimoxazole, two compound tablets twice daily *or*

Tetracycline 250 mg four times daily.

Amoxycillin is related to ampicillin and has very similar antibacterial effects. It is absorbed about twice as readily and seems likely to replace ampicillin in general use. In high dosage it is potentially bactericidal against *Haemophilus influenzae*. In severe exacerbations or where exacerbations occur frequently in a disabled subject a dose of 500 mg may be given six hourly for the first two days. This may eradicate *Haemophilus influenzae* from the sputum for some weeks.

DURATION OF TREATMENT

Antibiotic treatment should be continued until the sputum is again mucoid and for not less than five days. There is little evidence that long-term treatment with antibiotics is helpful.

4. Bronchodilator treatment

Oral bronchodilator preparations may bring about modest improvement in symptoms and are worthy of careful trial. Even slight amelioration of airways obstruction may be helpful in a disabled patient. There is no need for patients to take regular oral bronchodilators unless they can demonstrate benefit to their own satisfaction.

The use of aerosol bronchodilators usually produces more effective bronchodilatation. A salbutamol aerosol used in a dose of 2 puffs 4 times daily or as necessary up to 3 hourly may provide valuable relief.

5. Mucolytics

These agents play a minor role in the management of chronic bronchitis.

It is rare for patients to notice important symptomatic benefit. Brom-hexine in a dose of 16 mg four times daily may render sputum less tenacious and is worthy of trial in disabled patients who complain of excessive difficulty in producing viscid sputum.

6. Influenza prophylaxis

Disabled individuals should be immunised against expected epidemic strains of Influenza A virus.

Management of severely ill patients requiring admission to hospital

Management comprises:

a. Antibiotic therapy
b. Bronchodilator therapy
c. Encouragement to expectorate
d. Supervision of respiratory failure.

Parenteral antibiotic therapy may be necessary in desperately ill patients.

Intravenous bronchodilator therapy will be necessary in most instances. Aminophylline is effective and has stood the test of time. It may be given by continuous infusion or by slow intravenous injection over a few minutes. It causes respiratory stimulation, cardiac acceleration and frequently coughing and vomiting. It is desirable to follow intravenous aminophylline with vigorous encouragement to cough. Terbutaline causes less cardiac acceleration and may be given subcutaneously or intravenously as an alternative to aminophylline.

The majority of patients admitted to hospital with a severe exacerbation of chronic bronchitis accompanied by airways obstruction will recover in response to the above measures.

It may be difficult to decide whether or not the patient suffers from chronic asthma (p. 164). Where there is doubt in a severely ill individual it is reasonable to start intravenous or oral steroid therapy. The relevance of steroid therapy can be critically reviewed during the convalescent phase.

BASIC INVESTIGATIONS

1. *Chest X-ray*

Obvious pneumonia will affect antibiotic policy. There may be evidence of pneumothorax, pleural effusion, malignant disease etc., all of which may affect management from a quite early stage.

2. *Measurement of* P_{CO_2}
It is important to measure P_{CO_2} using arterial blood or rebreathing method at least once (p. 52).

3. *Measurement of* P_{O_2}
Very desirable if the patient is cyanosed.

4. *Blood urea and serum electrolytes*
Elevation of blood urea will suggest dehydration (common) or renal failure related to severe cardiac failure. Elevation of plasma bicarbonate level will suggest well-established chronic respiratory failure.

5. *Sputum culture*
This is particularly relevant when the patient is collapsed or pyrexial or has already failed to respond to adequate antibiotic therapy.

6. *Detailed documentation of disability*
Particular care should be taken to obtain details of the extent and duration of the patient's respiratory disability (and his tolerance of it) by interrogating close relatives at the time of admission. The extent to which the patient has been exposed to various forms of treatment should also be noted. If the patient deteriorates a decision on whether or not artificial ventilation should be undertaken cannot be made without this information.

Management of respiratory failure

Respiratory failure is generally regarded as being present when the arterial oxygen tension is low (in round figures below 9 kPa below 70 mmHg) and the arterial carbon dioxide tension is high (above 6·3 kPa or 47 mmHg). In exacerbations of chronic airways obstruction accompanying chronic bronchitis some degree of respiratory failure is common. Arterial P_{CO_2} is elevated because of reduced alveolar ventilation and arterial P_{O_2} is reduced partly as a direct consequence of the reduced alveolar ventilation and partly because of regional underventilation (ventilation-perfusion imbalance). Hypoxia is potentially lethal; hypercapnia is intoxicating but not immediately lethal.

THE PROBLEM OF OXYGEN THERAPY
Oxygen should not be given to patients in presumed respiratory failure without a good deal of careful thought; most patients do not need it.

Patients with established respiratory failure who have had a raised P_{CO_2} for some days become unresponsive to the CO_2 stimulus to ventilation and rely increasingly on hypoxia to maintain the drive to breathe. If they are given oxygen to breathe, they breathe less; if they are given high concentrations of oxygen, they breathe very much less. This underbreathing results in increasing hypercapnia which intoxicates and ultimately acts as a respiratory depressant. Oxygen should therefore logically be reserved for those patients with *severe hypoxia*. Unfortunately patients with severe hypoxia are generally those with a high PCO_2 and CO_2 insensitivity so that

> Patients who really need oxygen often cannot tolerate it and conversely
> Patients who tolerate oxygen often do not really need it.

Who has severe hypoxia?
This may be difficult to decide.

The severity of hypoxia depends largely upon:
Arterial oxygen content
Cardiac output
The distribution of the cardiac output (Fig. 23.1, p. 225).

The following points are worth making:

1 Patients in respiratory failure with cor pulmonale generally tolerate arterial hypoxaemia quite well since the cardiac output is usually normal.
2 Cyanosis is **not** an indication for oxygen therapy.
3 Severe hypoxia can be assumed to be present if the PO_2 is less than 4·7 kPa (35 mmHg).
4 There is some evidence that profuse sweating, moaning and grunting may denote severe hypoxia.

Controlled oxygen therapy
If oxygen is required it is required *continuously*. Intermittent oxygen is illogical and more dangerous than either continuous oxygen or no oxygen at all (see Chapter 23).

In established respiratory failure severe hypoxia should be treated initially with 24 per cent oxygen delivered by a venturi-type mask (Fig. 23.2); this may be enough to raise the arterial PO_2 to acceptable levels. However in severe cases the relief of hypoxia is followed by some fall in ventilation and the PO_2 falls to a level approaching that present before oxygen administration began. The aim is to increase the PO_2 *slightly* accepting that this may mean a *slight* rise in PCO_2. If high concentrations of oxygen are used then underventilation will be extreme before the hypoxic drive reappears.

The likely response to oxygen therapy can be judged from

1. *Level of PCO_2*. Above 9 kPa (or about 70 mmHg) underventilation will be a problem.

2. *The appearance of the patient*. If he looks as if he has a strong drive to breathe—he probably has (Fig. 16.1).

Underbreathing on oxygen may become evident within minutes but it may develop over hours or days with the patient becoming almost imperceptibly more somnolent and less inclined to clear his airways of accumulating sputum. Underbreathing on oxygen can be combated by measures to stimulate ventilation.

Respiratory stimulants

The most effective stimulant is regular encouragement to cough and take deep breaths which can be given by nurses, physiotherapists, relatives etc. The patient will generally breathe more effectively sitting up in bed or in a chair rather than curled up.

Nikethamide may be used intravenously in a dose of 2 ml (of 25 per cent solution) together with aminophylline up to 3 hourly followed by vigorous encouragement to produce sputum.

Doxapram is a useful short-acting respiratory stimulant which is given by continuous intravenous infusion in a dose of 1 to 2 mg per minute. It may be effective in combating the respiratory depressant effect of oxygen administration discussed above.

Treatment of heart failure

It is usual to digitalise patients with overt signs of cardiac failure although these signs usually subside without specific treatment once there is improvement in the respiratory failure. Frusemide appears to have a beneficial effect in established respiratory failure with or without oedema.

Avoidance of sedatives

Patients in severe respiratory failure with hypercapnia are frequently confused and very noisy. The temptation to use sedative drugs must be resisted. There is no sedative which does not aggravate hypoventilation.

Hypnotics should be avoided even between exacerbations in any patient who has shown a previous tendency to hypoventilation.

Arrested improvement

Occasional patients relapse after an initial period of improvement and they are found to have reached a state of equilibrium with a $P\text{CO}_2$ of about 10·5 kPa (80 mmHg or so). They are seen to be asleep much of the day perhaps having intermittent oxygen and apparently remaining too ill to be got out of bed. In addition to reintroducing treatment with aminophylline and nikethamide or doxapram the following measures may prove helpful: 1, administration of frusemide 80 or 120 mg twice daily; 2, complete withdrawal of oxygen; 3, venesection if the PCV is in excess of 53 per cent; 4, sitting the patient out of bed; 5, administration of the carbonic anhydrase inhibitor dichlorphenamide 50 mg three times daily. A proportion of patients will remain in chronic respiratory failure after recovery with a persistent elevation of $P\text{CO}_2$. The patient will usually be able to say when he is back to his usual state or better and this end-point should be heeded.

ARTIFICIAL VENTILATION

The use of intermittent positive pressure ventilation (IPPV) should be

considered when measures described so far fail to prevent deterioration and
1   It proves impossible to secure adequate oxygenation.
2   The patient is unable to cough up secretions through stupor or exhaustion.

Before embarking upon IPPV it is usual to review the patient's previous condition. If he has been totally immobilised and in misery despite adequate trial of available treatments it may not be kind to restore him temporarily to this existence. Once the decision has been taken to embark upon IPPV oxygen can be given continuously and endotracheal intubation carried out without undue delay by the most skilled person available. During IPPV the patient is sedated and rested and maintained on oxygen sufficient to keep the arterial Po_2 at about 60 mmHg. Secretions are removed by endobronchial suction. Vigorous mechanical ventilation is avoided because rapid lowering of the Pco_2 may lead to circulatory collapse. Large volumes of intravenous fluid and dextran are sometimes required at this stage to maintain adequate circulatory filling as judged by central venous pressure measurement. Usually at least 24 hours of IPPV is necessary. Attempts to withdraw ventilatory assistance are made on each following morning. Occasionally tracheostomy is necessary where recovery is slow and intermittent ventilatory assistance and tracheal suction continues to be required.

DOMICILIARY OXYGEN THERAPY See p. 231.

OTHER CAUSES OF
VENTILATORY FAILURE

Chronic bronchitis with airways obstruction is overwhelmingly the commonest cause of chronic ventilatory failure. A few patients with chronic severe asthma may develop chronic hypoventilation but other causes are rare.

Primary alveolar hypoventilation

This condition is apparently due to a central failure of respiratory drive. A proportion of individuals are obese and to this group the name 'Pickwickian' has been applied.

The condition may present with oedema, headache, somnolence and cyanosis. The provisional diagnosis is usually of obscure heart failure; there may be electrocardiographic and radiographic evidence of right ventricular hypertrophy. The arterial Pco_2 is always elevated and ventilatory tests yield normal results. Careful investigation of non-obese individuals may sometimes reveal evidence of bronchiectasis or of small airways narrowing. Patients with this condition show almost no ventilatory response to inhaled CO_2 despite good ventilatory function. They are able to exercise surprisingly well.

Restriction of chest wall movement

KYPHOSCOLIOSIS
Progressive ventilatory failure commonly accompanies severe kyphoscoliosis. In patients who also have chronic bronchitis ventilatory failure tends to appear even though the deformity may be relatively mild.

OTHER CONDITIONS
Ankylosing spondylitis and other conditions which limit chest movement may cause ventilatory failure. Progressive muscular weakness may have similar effects.

CHAPTER 17 · CARCINOMA OF THE BRONCHUS

Incidence

About 35,000 people die from carcinoma of the bronchus in the U.K. each year. Half of these deaths occur before the age of 65. The incidence has risen progressively since the beginning of the century—partly because it was frequently misdiagnosed as tuberculosis in earlier years but probably largely because of the increase in smoking. It is about 5 times more common in men than women. The rate of increase in mortality rate for men is slowing down but that for women continues to accelerate; women are catching up.

Aetiology

SMOKING

There is now an overwhelming body of evidence which indicates that cigarette smoking is the major cause of bronchial carcinoma:

1　The rise in deaths from carcinoma of the bronchus has reflected increasing exposure to cigarette smoking over the past 50 years particularly when the two sexes are studied separately.

2　The risk of death from bronchial carcinoma increases by a factor roughly equal to the number of cigarettes smoked per day. That is to say that an individual smoking 25 cigarettes daily has about 25 times greater chance of dying from the disease than a non-smoker of the same age and sex.

3　The risk of bronchial carcinoma is greatest in those who inhale cigarette smoke.

4　The risk of dying from bronchial carcinoma falls off dramatically if cigarette smoking stops. (The excess risk is approximately halved every 5 years after stopping smoking.) Pipe and cigar smokers have a small increased risk of bronchial carcinoma which is very much smaller than that of cigarette smokers.

OTHER FACTORS

The strength of the association between cigarette smoking and bronchial carcinoma tends to swamp other factors.

Urbanisation

The incidence of bronchial carcinoma is greater in urban than in rural areas, even when cigarette smoking is allowed for. Atmospheric pollution is regarded as the most likely explanation of this difference but the relationship is poorly defined.

Occupational factors

Occupational factors appear to play a relatively small part in the causation of the disease but there is nevertheless good evidence that industrial exposure to chromates, nickel, arsenic, coal gas and radioactive gases is associated with an increased risk of bronchial carcinoma. Carcinoma of the bronchus may complicate established asbestosis (p. 222).

Pathology

CELL TYPES

Four main types of carcinoma may be distinguished (Fig. 17.1). Sometimes histological classification proves difficult. The cell type has some relationship to the pattern of growth and response to treatment. Squamous cell carcinomas tend to grow more slowly and metastasise later than the other varieties. Adenocarcinomas appear not to be related to smoking exposure. The prognosis is worst with oat cell and anaplastic (undifferentiated) carcinoma.

SITE OF ORIGIN AND SPREAD

The majority of carcinomata originate in the larger bronchi and about two-thirds are visible on bronchoscopy (p. 180). The tumours spread by direct invasion of the lung, chest wall and mediastinal structures and particularly by metastasis to the hilar and the mediastinal lymph nodes.

Blood-borne distant metastasis is common; liver, adrenal gland and brain being particularly favoured organs. At death metastases are present in the great majority of cases.

Diagnosis

CLINICAL FEATURES

Bronchial carcinoma presents in a wide variety of ways. Commonly there are symptoms and clinical features relating to the chest but the disease may present with metastatic complications or non-metastatic neuro-endocrine syndromes or because of non-specific symptoms such as malaise and weight loss.

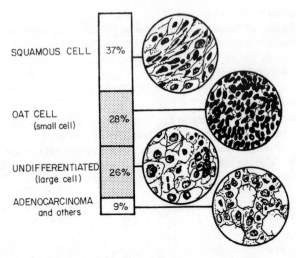

Fig. 17.1. *Histological types of bronchial carcinoma*
The percentages are approximate. Oat cell and undifferentiated large cell
carcinoma are sometimes grouped together in a single 'undifferentiated' or
'anaplastic' category. Typing is often difficult owing to variation in histological
appearances between different parts of the same tumour.

Chest symptoms

Cough. Chronic bronchitis is usually present anyway but a persistent
aggravation of cough may be the first feature of carcinoma.

Dyspnoea. Usually this is a late symptom due to collapse of an obstructed lobe or lung, pleural effusion or extensive lymphatic infiltration of
the lung.

Haemoptysis is common at any stage of the disease and occasionally
massive.

Chest pain. Very common. Sometimes diffuse and poorly localised but
tending to be constant. Sometimes well localised and related to chest wall
involvement. Central chest pain may be related to mediastinal gland enlargement.

Hoarseness when it is persistent may be due to involvement of the left
recurrent laryngeal nerve by hilar extension of the tumour. (Sometimes
unilateral laryngeal paralysis is asymptomatic.)

Chest signs
Commonly there may be no physical signs on examination of the chest.
Lymph node enlargement.
Signs of collapse (p. 42).
Signs of consolidation (p. 41).

Signs of pleural effusion (p. 42).

A particularly characteristic and sinister sign is *stridor* (p. 35) which usually reflects extensive involvement of a main bronchus or the trachea.

Clinical situations

Carcinoma is strongly suspected in cases of unresolved pneumonia or recurrent pneumonia and pleural effusion (especially if large, recurrent or bloodstained). There is an increased incidence of bronchial carcinoma in conditions causing diffuse pulmonary fibrosis (p. 140).

Metastatic complications

The range of syndromes encountered is large and includes cerebral tumour, paraplegia, painful hepatomegaly, obstructive jaundice, pathological fractures and bone pain, skin nodules etc., etc. Some syndromes deserve particular mention.

Superior vena caval obstruction

(Superior mediastinal syndrome.) This causes venous engorgement of the upper part of the body with facial congestion, oedema and headache particularly in the morning. Examination reveals a suffused facies and static, filled jugular veins with distension of the veins of the chest and upper limbs. Fine veins around the chest just above the costal margin are prominent and major collateral veins may be seen running down the axillae. S.V.C. obstruction is particularly likely to complicate carcinoma near the right hilum. These cases are inoperable but improvement may be produced by radiotherapy (p. 185).

Pancoasts's tumour

This term refers to carcinoma which extends upwards from the apex of the lung to invade the structures of the axilla. The lower part of the brachial plexus is particularly likely to be involved and this produces distressing pain down the inner surface of the arm. + bone destruction.

Horner's syndrome

Involvement of the sympathetic ganglia or the thoracic sympathetic fibres may result in the production of Horner's syndrome.

NON-METASTATIC EXTRA-PULMONARY MANIFESTATIONS

With the exception of clubbing, these manifestations are uncommon.

Endocrine disturbances

Hypercalcaemia. Of obscure causation; causes polyuria.

Inappropriate A.D.H. secretion. This usually presents with stupor, acute confusion or psychosis, sometimes accompanied by epilepsy. The feature may fluctuate. Some patients are misdiagnosed as suffering from intracranial metastases. A cardinal feature is the very low serum sodium level.

Cushing's disease. Bronchial carcinomas may be the site of inappropriate A.C.T.H. secretion.

Melanosis.

Gynaecomastia.

Neurological disturbances
  Diffuse encephalopathy.
  Cerebellar degeneration.
  Myelitis.
  Peripheral neuritis.
  Myasthenic syndrome.
  Polymyositis producing proximal weakness and wasting particularly of the trunk muscles.
  Dermatomyositis polymyositis with a violaceous telangectatic skin eruption.

These neurological features sometimes appear before there is any evidence of the bronchial carcinoma. They may regress after removal of the tumour.

Thrombophlebitis migrans

Bronchial carcinoma may present like other malignancies with repeated multiple peripheral venous thrombosis. Thrombosis in an upper limb is always suspicious.

Hypertrophic pulmonary osteoarthropathy

This is a rare complication. It presents with dull aching and sometimes swelling of the wrists or ankles. X-rays of the ends of the radius or tibia reveal subperiosteal new bone formation in the form of linear opacities parallel to the outer surface of the bone. Usually it is associated with advanced clubbing. Other disorders which cause clubbing may rarely cause hypertrophic pulmonary osteoarthropathy.

RADIOLOGICAL FEATURES

The chest X-ray usually provides the most compelling early evidence of bronchial carcinoma. A wide range of appearances is encountered.

Rounded shadow

This is the most common X-ray finding at the time of presentation. Usually it is already in excess of 2 cm in diameter and may have a fluffy or spiked appearance at its border or there may be radially arranged shadows indicating infiltration or patchy collapse peripheral to the mass. Slower-growing squamous carcinomata may have a relatively smooth contour. Cavitation within the rounded shadow is common. Occasionally the carcinoma is a tiny nodule when first seen.

Collapse of a lobe or lung
In smoking adults this finding is most usually due to carcinoma of the bronchus although there are of course many other possible causes.

Hilar or mediastinal enlargement
These changes are usually the result of lymph node metastases.

Pleural effusion
Particularly if it is large or accompanied by other features outlined above always raises the possibility of bronchial carcinoma.

Lymphangitis carcinomatosa
This term refers to diffuse spread of carcinoma through the lymphatic channels of the lungs. Carcinomas of various types particularly adeno-carcinomata of stomach and breast may present this picture particularly after mediastinal involvement. There is usually fairly severe dyspnoea. The X-ray appearances are of streaky micronodular mottling which is generally radially arranged and which may be very widespread. When bronchial carcinoma is the cause the shadowing is usually asymmetrical and there may be a solid lesion. Localised streaky shadowing suggestive of lymphatic obstruction or infiltration is common in the immediate neighbourhood of bronchial carcinomata.

No abnormality
The chest X-ray is found to be normal in only a small proportion of patients. In these the lesion is either very tiny (in cases presenting perhaps with remote metastatic or non-metastatic syndromes) or it is situated proximally in main bronchus or trachea.

Tomography
Sometimes better visualisation of a lesion is possible with this technique. Narrowing of the trachea or main bronchus may be revealed. Tomography is expensive, rarely furthers the diagnosis appreciably and it should not be regarded as obligatory when a localised abnormality is detected on plain films.

Bronchography
This may occasionally be useful particularly in localising tumours prior to surgery.

HISTOLOGICAL/CYTOLOGICAL CONFIRMATION
The diagnosis may be near-certain from clinical and radiological features alone but an attempt should normally be made to obtain histological or cytological confirmation.

Sputum cytology

The diagnostic yield from cytological examination depends upon the experience and interest of the pathology service and upon the provision of adequate fresh specimens of true sputum. In about half of patients with advanced bronchial carcinoma diagnostic appearances are evident if at least 3 good specimens are examined. The yield in small peripheral lesions is very low.

Bronchoscopy

Bronchoscopy is usually indicated in suspected bronchial carcinoma. The aim is (a) to obtain histological confirmation of the diagnosis and (b) to assess operability. About two-thirds of tumours can be seen at bronchoscopy and biopsied. The recent introduction of the fibre-optic bronchoscope has increased this figure especially in the case of upper-lobe tumours which are particularly difficult to inspect and biopsy with the standard rigid instrument. Bronchoscopy may be omitted in superior vena caval obstruction and in terminal cases where there is no possibility of surgical treatment and the diagnosis has already been obtained by cytological or other measures. Rigid bronchoscopy is generally carried out under general anaesthesia with intravenous agents and muscle relaxants (Fig. 17.2).

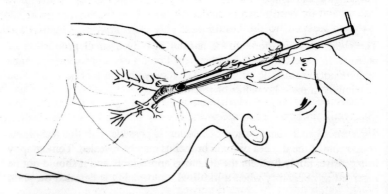

Fig. 17.2. *Bronchoscopy using a rigid bronchoscope*
Depending upon its size, the instrument can be passed most of the way down the main bronchi. Views of the orifices of the segmental bronchi are obtained (with the aid of angled telescopes in the case of the upper lobes). Rather less of the bronchial tree than is shown in the diagram is available for inspection.

Ventilation is maintained by venturi entrainment of air with a nozzle injecting high-pressure oxygen at intervals into the bronchoscope.

The fibre-optic bronchoscope is now widely used in diagnosis, sometimes passed through a rigid instrument but more usually introduced transnasally in the conscious seated patient using topical anaesthesia. It is convenient, causes minimal upset to the patient and permits improved visualisation particularly of the upper lobes.

The following findings all suggest that the lesion may be inoperable: Involvement of the proximal part of a main bronchus particularly the left. Widening of the carina or tracheal compression from mediastinal lymph nodes and left vocal cord paralysis due to left recurrent laryngeal nerve involvement.

Needle biopsy
Aspiration needle biopsy may produce diagnostically useful cytological material from peripheral solid tumours. If such lesions are large a Vim-Silverman needle can be used. A trephine biopsy may be used in diffuse lung involvement.

In the case of smaller peripheral shadows there may be no need to persist with attempts to obtain histology because an early thoracotomy is almost always indicated if pulmonary function permits. Carcinoma is the commonest cause of small rounded shadows and this group has the best chance of successful surgical treatment.

Pleural aspiration
When there is an effusion valuable evidence may be obtained from the cytological content of the fluid. It is desirable to get the patient to roll about and tip head down immediately prior to aspiration otherwise cells tend to sediment to the bottom and only clear fluid may be aspirated. Pleural biopsy should always be carried out.

Pleural biopsy
The usual technique employs the Abrams punch (Fig. 17.3). This is introduced into the pleural space under local anaesthetic. Where the pleura is greatly thickened good specimens may be obtained with the air-driven trephine.

Mediastinoscopy and scalene-node biopsy
Mediastinoscopy comprises inspection of mediastinal structures, particularly lymph nodes by blunt dissection downwards from the suprasternal notch sometimes using a modified laryngoscope. Biopsy of mediastinal nodes may provide confirmation of the diagnosis (and of inoperability) prior to radiotherapeutic treatment particularly when bronchoscopy is negative despite obvious mediastinal or hilar enlargement. Scalene-node

biopsy may be performed with the same aim. These techniques are useful when Hodgkin's disease, lymphosarcoma or occasionally sarcoidosis are likely alternative diagnoses.

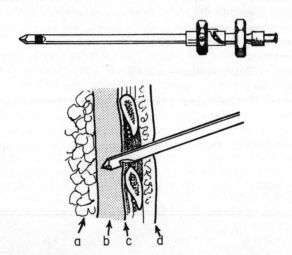

Fig. 17.3. *Pleural biopsy using the Abrams punch*
The instrument is in two parts. The outer pointed sheath has a notch near the tip and carries a spiral groove at the proximal end. The inner cylinder has a sharp cutting edge at its distal end and a lateral peg at its proximal end which fits into the spiral groove. When the two parts of the instrument are rotated relative to each other the spiral groove causes the inner cutting cylinder to close the notch cutting off any tissue engaged in its mouth.

Below the instrument is shown in position for obtaining a pleural biopsy. After aspirating fluid the instrument is withdrawn until the notch snags on the pleural surface. The cutting edge is then rotated into the closed position and the instrument withdrawn. (a) lung; (b) pleural fluid; (c) parietal pleura; (d) skin surface.

Liver biopsy

Where there is liver enlargement or jaundice liver biopsy may provide histological confirmation. The yield from this investigation can be improved by carrying out a *liver scan* and directing the biopsy needle to any accessible 'cold area' which is revealed.

Thoracotomy

The diagnosis may not be confirmed until thoracotomy is performed. Where all the evidence points to an operable bronchial carcinoma and there are no major contraindications, thoracotomy should not be unnecessarily delayed as the danger of metastasis increases with every day which passes.

Treatment

The options comprise:
1 Radical surgery
2 Palliative surgery
3 Radical radiotherapy
4 Palliative radiotherapy
5 Chemotherapy
6 Palliative medical and nursing measures
7 No treatment.

Each case will require careful individual consideration and the choice of treatment will be affected by such considerations as extent and type of the tumour, the age of the patient and presence of other (especially cardio-pulmonary) diseases, the nature of the symptoms and also upon the patient's wishes.

I. RADICAL SURGERY

This offers the best chance of long-term survival in suitable cases where the tumour is apparently well localised to a lobe or a lung and the patient can tolerate the excision. Unfortunately half of the patients with bacterial carcinoma are unsuitable for resection because of obvious spread to the mediastinum or beyond or because of coexistent cardiopulmonary disability. Of those who are operated upon half are found to have unresectable disease. Of those in whom the tumour is apparently resected at operation about 25 per cent are still alive at 5 years (Fig. 17.4). The operative mortality is generally 15 to 20 per cent depending upon how aggressive the selection policy is.

Preoperative functional assessment

Chronic bronchitis and associated airways obstruction frequently accompany bronchial carcinoma and may make resection impossible. No single test permits prediction of feasibility of pneumonectomy and the decision depends on the balance of clinical and laboratory evidence taken in conjunction with the likelihood of successful removal of tumour. Greater risks are justified in the case of a small squamous cell carcinoma.

The following features are associated with a high mortality and intolerable disability after pneumonectomy. An FEV_1 of less than half the predicted value, single-breath transfer factor of less than half the predicted value and evidence of chronic respiratory failure (elevated Pco_2). Exercise dyspnoea of Grade II or worse.

2. PALLIATIVE SURGERY

This is rarely carried out but it may be useful in Pancoast's tumour where severe pain results from involvement of the brachial plexus or in the management of broncho-pleural fistula, severe haemoptysis etc. Various neurosurgical procedures such as tractotomy and thalamectomy may be occasionally indicated for terrible pain from other areas.

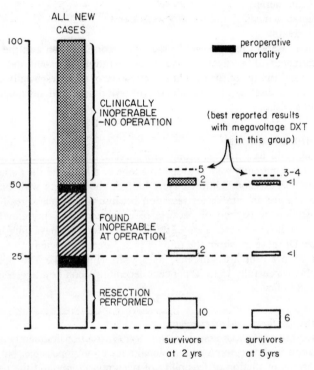

Fig. 17.4. *Operability and survival in bronchial carcinoma*
The figures are approximate and no account is taken of histological type.

3. RADICAL RADIOTHERAPY

The advent of megavoltage techniques has allowed larger doses to be given in a shorter time and with relatively less unwanted tissue damage. Various techniques exist; most aim at a total dose of 4,000–6,000 rads over the course of 3 to 4 weeks. The use of modern megavoltage techniques has increased the effectiveness of radiotherapy in recent years and in some circumstances the results are better than those following surgery.

RADICAL SURGERY OR RADICAL RADIOTHERAPY?

(i) Clinically operable cases

Small-cell (oat cell) tumours do badly however treated but radiotherapy may produce slightly better results than surgery. Squamous cell carcinomas survive better after surgical removal than after radiotherapy.

(ii) Clinically inoperable cases

Survival has been improved with megavoltage radiotherapy in inoperable bronchial carcinoma confined to the thorax. Mean 3-year survival is about 10 per cent in squamous carcinoma and adenocarcinoma and 4 per cent in the case of anaplastic and oat cell tumours.

4. PALLIATIVE RADIOTHERAPY

This is undertaken for the relief of symptoms. A particular indication for palliative treatment is the presence of superior vena caval obstruction. The obstruction generally subsides dramatically after a few days and usually it does not recur as the disease progresses. Pain due to chest wall invasion or bone metastases may be susceptible to radiotherapy.

5. CHEMOTHERAPY

Cytotoxic drugs have a very limited place in the palliative management of bronchial carcinoma. Careful trials of combinations of chemotherapeutic agents give some cause for hope that survival in small-cell carcinoma may in time be usefully extended.

In a rapidly recurring pleural effusion it is sometimes possible to avert the reaccumulation of fluid by weekly aspiration and insertion of mustine derivatives (e.g. triethylene thiophosphoramide 15 mg). Temporary control of superior venacaval obstruction may be obtained with i.v. treatment where there are no readily available facilities for radiotherapy.

6. PALLIATIVE MEDICAL AND NURSING MEASURES

The patient's principal need from his medical and nursing attendants is their time. There is great scope for alert symptomatic treatment in progressive bronchial carcinoma particularly in connection with cough (which usually responds to methadone linctus if necessary in large doses) and pain which may require strong analgesics. Where wasting and anorexia are themselves the focus of distress it is worth prescribing a modest dose of oral steroids. In the terminal stages if anxiety, pain and dyspnoea are prominent *regular* injections of diamorphine are usually the most reliable means of producing calm and equanimity without undue sedation.

7. NO TREATMENT

In very old or disabled individuals with few symptoms the discovery of inoperable carcinoma does not usually demand any treatment.

Alveolar cell carcinoma

This rather uncommon tumour arises from alveolar or bronchiolar epithelium and spreads along the alveolar and bronchiolar surfaces. The affected areas tend to become filled with whorls of tumour cells but the essential architecture of the lung parenchyma is preserved in the early stages at least. The tumour presents with cough, haemoptysis or non-specific symptoms. The chest X-ray may show irregular rounded or shaggy shadows which are unevenly distributed in one lobe or lung. The tumour sometimes appears to be disseminated or perhaps multi-focal in origin. Misdiagnosis is common (most usually as tuberculosis) and the correct diagnosis may only be made at thoracotomy. Cytological examination of the sputum is sometimes helpful. The tumour is sometimes slow growing and in localised tumours the results of surgery are appreciably better than for bronchial carcinoma. Diffuse tumours do not respond to radiotherapy and are always fatal.

Bronchial adenoma

These uncommon tumours normally present with haemoptysis, cough and sputum and sometimes there is bronchial obstruction with distal collapse. Half may be biopsied at bronchoscopy. The great majority are bronchial carcinoids which are slow growing, locally invasive and which only rarely metastasise. Clinical evidence of secretory activity—the carcinoid syndrome —is rare and suggests the presence of metastases. The majority of the remaining tumours are cylindromata. These tumours are also slow growing and locally invasive but at least 10 per cent show malignant features. The overall mortality amongst patients with bronchial adenoma is of the order of 10 per cent. If there are no metastases evident at the time of the operation and histological examination reveals no atypical features, long-term survival is the rule.

Mesothelioma (See p. 223.)

CHAPTER 18 · PULMONARY EMBOLISM AND PULMONARY HYPERTENSION

PULMONARY EMBOLISM

Pulmonary embolism is **important** in that it is potentially fatal, often preventable and sometimes treatable. The mode of presentation depends to a large extent on the size of the embolus (Fig. 18.1).

Source

Thrombosis—the systemic veins and occasionally the right side of the heart is the usual source of emboli.

VENOUS THROMBOSIS
A number of factors predispose to venous thrombosis.

1 *Damage to vein wall* due to local trauma or inflammation.

2 *Slowing of the circulation*—immobility, local pressure, venous obstruction, varicose veins, congestive cardiac failure, shock, dehydration, hypovolaemia etc.

3 *Hypercoagulability of the blood.* Associated with recent trauma, childbirth or operations, thrombocythaemia, oral contraceptives, malignant disease etc.

Clinical evidence of venous thrombosis
Thrombosis in deep veins of the legs, pelvis or abdomen may be completely silent and be unsuspected until pulmonary embolism ensues (phlebothrombosis). The relative lack of local inflammatory reaction in the vessel wall may result in the clot being only loosely attached. Where there is more local inflammation of the vein (thrombophlebitis) the characteristic features of local *warmth*, tenderness, oedema and superficial venous dilatation are more evident and the clot may be more securely adherent. *The severity of the local signs is a relatively poor indication of the risk of pulmonary embolism.*

Confirmatory tests of venous thrombosis
1. *Ultrasonic probe.* Occlusion of major leg veins may be revealed by this means. An ultrasonic probe is placed over a major vein (popliteal or iliofemoral) and the calf or thigh distal to the probe is compressed. The probe

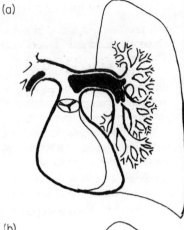

Fig. 18.1. *Synopis of pulmonary embolism*

(a) MASSIVE PULMONARY EMBOLISM
Sudden circulatory collapse
  Hypotension, unconsciousness, cold
  mottled periphery. Cyanosis.
Central chest pain
Hyperventilation
Engorged neck veins
E.C.G. Sometimes RV strain pattern
C.X.R. Usually unhelpful
Angio. Shows obstruction
Scan. Not done

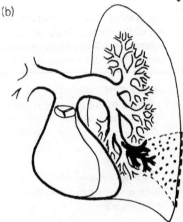

(b) MEDIUM-SIZED EMBOLI
With Infarction
  Pleural pain haemoptysis,
    effusion, fever, hyperventilation.
  C.X.R. Segmental collapse/consolidation.
Without Infarction
  May be 'silent'.
  ? dyspnoea, hyperventilation
  ? fever.
  C.X.R. may be normal
E.C.G. Unhelpful
Angio. Usually shows obstruction if early.
Scan. Usually reflects obstruction.

(c) REPEATED SMALL EMBOLI
Progressive breathlessness, hyperventilation
? effort syncope.
E.C.G. Right ventricular hypertrophy and
  axis deviation
C.X.R. Prominent pulmonary artery
Angio. May be normal or show slow circulation
  or peripheral 'pruning'
Scan Normal

will produce a signal if blood accelerates through the vein beneath and absence of the signal (generally an audible one) suggests venous occlusion. The test is crude but rapid and atraumatic.

2. *Venography*. Radiopaque contrast material is injected into a vein on the foot and films taken as it traverses the veins higher in the leg. This technique gives good evidence of major venous occlusion but is time consuming, expensive and moderately uncomfortable.

3. I^{125} *fibrinogen*. The isotope is injected intravenously and the uptake in the legs compared with the uptake in other regions of the body. Preferential uptake suggests the incorporation of the fibrinogen into fresh thrombus.

Clinical features, diagnosis and management

The consequences of pulmonary embolism depend very much upon the size of the emboli. Massive pulmonary embolism presents with circulatory collapse. Medium-sized pulmonary emboli tend to cause pulmonary infarction and a 'pneumonic' picture and multiple very small emboli cause gradual obstruction of the circulation and pulmonary hypertension leading to gradually progressive dyspnoea and right heart failure.

These broad categories will be discussed separately.

Massive pulmonary embolism

CLINICAL FEATURES

Massive pulmonary embolism causes its effects by suddenly plugging up the pulmonary circulation producing catastrophic drop in cardiac output. It presents with sudden collapse—the patient becomes shocked, pale and sweaty and usually strikingly tachypnoeic. Consciousness may be lost, usually transiently, and there may be fitting. The pulse is feeble and rapid and the blood pressure low, a third or fourth heart sound may be audible. The periphery becomes pale and cold and there may be mottled cyanosis especially in dependent areas. The cyanosis is generally central and may be unresponsive to oxygen administration. Where consciousness is preserved severe crushing chest pain may be present. The neck veins are usually strikingly engorged.

When the circulation is more or less completely arrested death ensues rapidly and the picture is that of a 'cardiac arrest' and ventricular fibrillation may in fact be present. In this desperate situation there is a notably poor response to external cardiac massage even when promptly applied.

DIAGNOSIS

This is commonly obvious from the circumstances (e.g. associated with postoperative venous thrombosis). The other conditions which often have to be considered are:

1. *Myocardial infarction.* Distinction may be difficult in the early stages especially (when typical E.C.G. changes of infarction might not have developed). Acute right bundle branch block and T-wave depression in V_1–4 suggest embolism but *the E.C.G. is often normal.* Excessive dyspnoea without signs of pulmonary oedema may suggest embolism.

2. *Acute internal blood loss.* The most helpful distinguishing feature is the state of the neck veins which will be barely filled even in the recumbent patient if blood loss is the explanation for profound collapse and well filled in acute massive embolism.

3. *Acute bacteraemic shock or pancreatitis.* Onset is generally less rapid, there may be evidence of the primary cause and central venous pressure will be low.

4. *Cardiac tamponade.* Tamponade due to pericardial effusion will generally appear more gradually, there may be paradoxical variation of venous (up in inspiration) and arterial (down in inspiration) pressures. Haemopericardium may be due to ruptured myocardial infarction, cardiac surgery trauma, pericarditis (especially on anticoagulants). Diagnosis of sudden tamponade may be difficult. The size of the heart shadow on a chest X-ray may be helpful.

5. *Dissecting aortic aneurysm* may mimic pulmonary embolism. Sometimes the chest X-ray shows widening of the aorta.

6. *Pneumothorax and massive collapse of a lung.* May produce sudden shock but will normally be identifiable by careful examination of the chest and by chest X-ray.

Where sudden death is averted there is usually some improvement in the patient's condition over minutes or hours attributable to movement of the clot further into one or both lungs.

CONFIRMATORY TESTS

The most satisfactory investigation is pulmonary arteriography which will usually demonstrate the obstructed zone. Lung scanning may be indicated if the patient's condition is good and there is serious doubt about the diagnosis. It is not normally carried out in this situation.

TREATMENT

1. *Emergency treatment* comprises the administration of oxygen; there is very little else that can be done.

2. *Fibrinolytic therapy.* Where the patient's condition continues to give cause for concern but he is considered likely to survive at least 24 hours fibrinolytic therapy is indicated. Streptokinase 600,000 units administered intravenously and an infusion continued for up to 72 hours. This treatment

provokes the thrombolytic mechanisms and greatly accelerates clearing of clot.

3. *Embolectomy* is now rarely carried out but may be necessary where the peripheral circulation fails to be restored after a few hours and hypotension persists. Angiography may be of some assistance in highlighting those individuals who require surgical treatment. Thrombolytic therapy has made embolectomy a rather rare measure.

4. *Anticoagulant treatment.* This is instituted after fibrinolytic therapy is complete.

PROGNOSIS

The prognosis is very variable but about 30 per cent of truly massive emboli prove fatal. The outlook is usually clear within a few hours of the onset and is obviously related to the rapidity of recovery. Commonly an acute massive embolus occurs on a background of several preceding emboli which may have blocked off much of the remaining pulmonary circulation. Anticoagulation reduces the risk of further embolism to about half.

Medium-sized pulmonary emboli

Usually embolisation presents with pleural pain perhaps accompanied by breathlessness, fever and cough productive of blood-streaked sputum. There may be signs of pleural effusion and a pleural rub or evidence of localised consolidation. Repeated medium-sized embolisation may occur relatively silently in recumbent ill patients particularly in the elderly. The only clinical feature may be tachypnoea.

The diagnosis depends upon thinking of pulmonary emboli whenever 'pneumonia' is the preliminary diagnosis. Aspiration of the pleural effusion usually yields a modest amount of blood-tinged fluid but sometimes the fluid is clear.

INVESTIGATIONS

The chest X-ray commonly shows elevation of the diaphragm with linear areas of atelectasis in the basal zones but may show no abnormality. The appearances of bilateral basal shadowing in a breathless patient should always suggest pulmonary embolism if no other cause is evident.

Pulmonary function tests

Nearly always the patient is found to be hyperventilating and the $P\text{co}_2$ is low. Other tests of pulmonary function are not very helpful—there may be increased deadspace ventilation but this is tedious to measure, the normal range is very wide and it is found to be increased in many forms of pulmonary disorder.

The lung scan

Technique. Macroaggregated human albumin is labelled with a gamma-emitting radioisotope (generally Technetium 99^m) and a dose is injected intravenously. The particles of the preparation are of such a size that they impact in pulmonary capillaries. (Only about 1 in 1,000 capillaries are obstructed and no detectable harm results. The albumin particles are broken down after a few hours.) A scintillation counting head passes to and fro across the chest and a printer attached to it prints marks on a piece of paper as gamma rays are detected—building up a life-size pattern of the distribution of the isotope alternatively a gamma camera may be employed. The result is a perfusion scan—it indicates the distribution of pulmonary blood flow.

Uses. 'Cold areas' are evident on the scan wherever there is a large area of defective blood flow and this is obviously useful in supporting a diagnosis of pulmonary embolism. Other localised conditions of the lung such as pneumonia or carcinoma are associated with localised defects of perfusion. The lung scan does not differentiate between embolism and other causes of defective perfusion associated with obvious radiological abnormality. It is however more useful if it demonstrates defective perfusion in areas which are not the site of obvious collapse or consolidation on the chest X-ray (Fig. 18.2).

In summary the evidence which lung scans produce concerning distribution of perfusion must be interpreted in the light of the chest X-ray appearances and the clinical circumstances.

Pulmonary arteriography

If performed within a few days pulmonary arteriography will usually demonstrate embolised zones if they are large enough. The extent to which these investigations are employed in providing confirmation of the diagnosis depends upon the extent to which the diagnosis is in doubt and also upon the condition of the patient. For example arteriography and lung scanning can hardly be regarded as essential to confirm clinically obvious embolism in the post-operative period or in association with manifest leg vein thrombosis. On the other hand in a patient being treated for bleeding peptic ulcer it would be important to have the advantage of all the evidence available from special investigations to be absolutely certain that embolism *was* occurring before embarking upon anticoagulant therapy which would carry substantial hazard in these circumstances.

TREATMENT

Immediate

Measures to relieve pain are required in the early stage when pleurisy may be extremely distressing. Opiate drugs are most useful. Anticoagulation is usually obligatory. If the patient is breathless and there are signs of extensive embolism, fibrinolytic therapy may be employed before anti-coagulation.

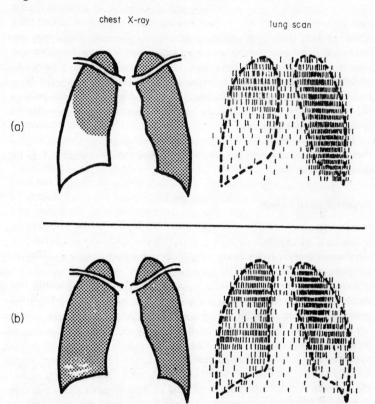

chest X-ray   lung scan

(a)

(b)

Fig. 18.2. (a) Chest X-ray and lung scan in a patient with a large right-sided pleural effusion. The lung scan shows normal perfusion on the left side and defective perfusion on the right such as might be expected in the presence of a pleural effusion or other obvious localised lung disease. In this case the lung scan has contributed no additional information.

(b) Chest X-ray shows minor linear shadowing at the right base but the lung scan shows large 'cold' areas in both lungs indicating impaired perfusion in these zones. The changes evident on the lung scan are out of proportion to those seen on the chest X-ray and in this case the lung scan has provided important additional information (which is strongly suggestive of pulmonary embolism).

Long-term—how long should anticoagulants be continued?
Where embolism occurs in the postoperative period or in association with an acute thrombophlebitis an arbitrary period of 2–3 months is usually sufficient. Where there is repeated embolism with either long-established

venous disorder or with no obvious primary site for thrombosis it may be necessary to continue anticoagulants indefinitely.

PROGNOSIS

Anticoagulant therapy is generally effective in preventing new thrombus formation but further embolism from existing clot is always possible for several days after starting treatment. Usually healing of the lung is near-complete, the affected areas re-expand or contract to linear scars. Sometimes pleural adhesions produce lingering painful tethering of the chest and the vital capacity may be slightly reduced. Haemoptysis sometimes continues for a week or more.

If numerous repeated medium-sized emboli occur, significant obstruction to the pulmonary circulation and pulmonary hypertension may develop (see below).

Repeated small emboli

CLINICAL FEATURES

Very small emboli (microemboli) will go unnoticed until a large part of the pulmonary circulation has become impacted. If repeated embolisation continues over weeks or months pulmonary hypertension develops. The outstanding symptom is dyspnoea on exercise which is generally an easy, panting dyspnoea resembling that seen in cardiac disease. Severe pulmonary hypertension is eventually accompanied by clinical E.C.G. and radiological evidence of right ventricular hypertrophy (Fig. 18.3). Tiredness, syncope on effort and angina reflect a critically limited cardiac output. Usually there is no obvious peripheral source of emboli although many of the patients with this disorder are found to have extensive varicose veins. A proportion of the remainder may follow pregnancy or use of oral contraceptive agents. Rarely tumour emboli (e.g. trophoblastic tumours or carcinoma of the breast) may lead to the appearance of pulmonary hypertension.

INVESTIGATIONS

Electrocardiogram
This will generally show clear evidence of right ventricular hypertrophy (Fig. 18.3 and p. 197).

The chest X-ray
This will generally reveal prominence of the pulmonary arterial conus and proximal pulmonary arteries; there may be a suggestion of under-vascularisation of the peripheral lung fields.

Pulmonary arteriography
This is generally unhelpful and merely shows dilated proximal pulmonary arteries and a rather slow pulmonary circulation.

Lung scanning
This is similarly unhelpful. There may be relatively poor perfusion of the bases but by the time severe symptoms are present the whole of the pulmonary circulation is involved and regional underperfusion is not seen.

Cardiac catheterisation
This is important—1, the presence of pulmonary hypertension is confirmed; 2, by measuring wedge pressure, left heart disease (particularly unsuspected mitral stenosis) is excluded; 3, by measuring the oxygen content of the blood in the right heart, a left to right shunt may be excluded.

TREATMENT
Long-term anticoagulant treatment is the only really important treatment apart from anti-failure measures where they are necessary.

PROGNOSIS
The outlook depends upon severity and duration but is generally poor. Once established, pulmonary hypertension is usually progressive. Patients who lack an obvious source for pulmonary emboli fall into the group labelled idiopathic primary pulmonary hypertension.

IDIOPATHIC PRIMARY
PULMONARY HYPERTENSION

This rare disorder presents in precisely the same manner as microthrombo-embolic pulmonary hypertension and usually the cause is unknown. In 1957–9 a large number of cases appeared in central Europe which seemed to be related to consumption of aminorex fumarate—an anorectic agent used to assist weight loss.

The course is almost always progressive and the disease is fatal within a few months or years. Exceptional individuals survive 10 years. Death either occurs suddenly, probably from syncope, or gradually with intractable heart failure. Anticoagulants are generally used because it is virtually impossible to exclude microthromboembolism. Vasodilation such as tolazoline (Priscol) may provide some relief and Persantin may help, perhaps by exerting an effect upon platelet function.

COR PULMONALE

Some confusion arises from the differing ways in which this term is employed. Essentially it means heart disease secondary to primary disease of the lungs. Some (particularly American) clinicians use the term to indicate any cardiac change—especially E.C.G. evidence of right ventricular hypertrophy. Others reserve the term to describe episodes of overt heart failure especially those which accompany chronic airways obstruction with respiratory failure. Pulmonary embolism is not usually included in the group labelled cor pulmonale.

In practice persons who develop right-sided heart disease have chronic hypoxia in common. In persons with airways obstruction cor pulmonale (however defined) is confined to individuals who are chronically hypoventilating and have elevated levels of arterial PCO_2 as well as hypoxia. In diffuse parenchymal disorders such as fibrosing alveolitis cor pulmonale develops at a late stage when there is chronic hypoxia. In this instance the patient is usually not underventilating and the PCO_2 is normal or low until terminally.

Hypoxia is of course a potent cause of pulmonary arteriolar constriction.

Evidence of right ventricular hypertrophy

CLINICAL

1 In the absence of airways obstruction the signs comprise a prominent parasternal heave, a loud pulmonary second sound (the last component of a split-second sound on inspiration) and sometimes a right atrial protodiastolic gallop. In very severe pulmonary hypertension pulmonary valve incompetence and tricuspid incompetence may supervene.

2 Where pulmonary hypertension is secondary to obstructive airways disease right ventricular hypertrophy is difficult to diagnose clinically because overinflation of the chest almost invariably obscures the physical signs.

THE E.C.G. (letters in brackets refer to Fig. 18.3)
The best evidence is provided by the chest leads—other features merely provide helpful support.

1. Leads V_1-2
The appearance of a QR complex or an RSR' complex in which the R' is bigger than the initial R constitutes strong evidence of right ventricular hypertrophy (a). Widening of the QRS complex is also suggestive; the T wave is commonly inverted (b).

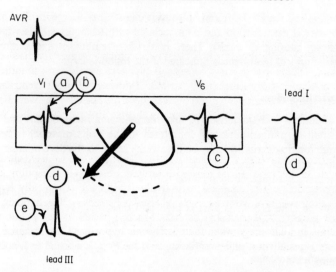

Fig. 18.3. *E.C.G. changes in right ventricular hypertrophy*
The solid arrow represents the mean QRS vector in the frontal plane; it is deflected to the right as indicated by the interrupted arrow. See text for description.

2. *Lateral chest leads* (V_5–V_6)

Deep S waves suggest right ventricular hypertrophy (c). Usually this is accompanied by 'clockwise rotation' with the QRS complex becoming mainly positive only in V_5 or V_6 (V_3 or V_4 in the normal).

3. *Other supporting evidence*

This may take the form of *right axis deviation* (a mean QRS vector in the frontal plane of greater than 100°—crudely detected by observing the dominant QRS to be directed downwards in lead I and upwards in lead III (d) 'pointing towards each other'). ST depression and T-wave inversion may be present in the inferior leads (II, III, VF). Right atrial hypertrophy may be reflected by *P. pulmonale*—tall peaked P waves with a vertical axis best seen in inferior leads (e).

SOME UNCOMMON CONDITIONS AFFECTING PULMONARY VASCULATURE

Pulmonary arteriovenous aneurysm (arteriovenous fistula)

The lesion takes the form of a lobulated swelling connecting pulmonary artery and pulmonary vein. Small or medium-sized fistulae produce no symptoms and tend to be found on routine chest X-ray. Large fistulae may cause arterial desaturation and be associated with telangectasia elsewhere (e.g. nose, causing epistaxis). There is a risk of embolism and cerebral abscess. Surgical treatment is indicated if the lesion is large.

Polyarteritis nodosa

This condition is characterised by arteritic lesions in many organs due to deposition of antigen-antibody complexes in the walls of small vessels. The pulmonary circulation may be involved leading to the development of multiple nodular infarcts which may be evident on the chest X-ray. Polyarteritis is sometimes associated with asthma. The diagnosis becomes evident by virtue of associated arteritic lesions in the skin, kidney or nervous tissue. The E.S.R. is always high and there may be blood eosinophilia. Treatment with corticosteroids is indicated.

Wegener's granuloma

This rare condition is generally regarded as a variant of polyarteritis nodosa. The principal features are: 1, nasal or aural granulomata causing ulceration, crusting, pain and bone erosion; 2, pulmonary nodules 0·5–1·5 cm in diameter; 3, renal involvement. The diagnosis may be made from the features described and supported by biopsy. The condition was formerly invariably fatal but prolonged survival is regularly achieved with corticosteroid and immunosuppressive drugs.

Goodpasture's syndrome

The combination of glomerulonephritis and intra-alveolar haemorrhage is called Goodpasture's syndrome. Haemoptysis may be striking or slight and mottling is generally evident on the chest X-ray. The pulmonary lesion may precede the onset of nephritis. Differentiation from polyarteritis nodosa depends on whether there is evidence of arteritis in other areas apart from the kidneys. The distinction may be artificial. The associated glomerulonephritis is generally very severe.

Idiopathic pulmonary haemosiderosis

This rare condition is characterised by repeated intra-alveolar capillary haemorrhage of obscure cause. It presents in childhood or young adult life with either anaemia or haemoptysis. The chest X-ray generally shows a miliary mottling pattern. The diagnosis may be confirmed by lung biopsy. Treatment with corticosteroids is generally tried but may have little effect. Death may follow a massive haemoptysis.

CHAPTER 19 · PULMONARY OEDEMA

In its simplest terms pulmonary oedema may be regarded as an increase in the fluid content of the extravascular tissues of the lung. Pulmonary oedema may result from reflex neurogenic mechanisms which are very poorly understood (e.g. in association with head injury or intracerebral tumour or haemorrhage) and alveolar oedema may follow interference with the normal functioning of the pulmonary capillaries and alveolar lining cells as occurs in poisoning with certain gases but the commonest cause of pulmonary oedema is increased capillary pressure due to impaired performance of the left heart.

PRIMITIVE VIEW OF PULMONARY OEDEMA

Until fairly recently the prevailing view of pulmonary oedema was that increased capillary filtration led immediately to fluid entering the alveoli and that this fluid then caused bubbling sounds (crepitations). This simple model ignores the important effects of the interstitial space and the function of lymphatic channels.

INTERSTITIAL OEDEMA

Electron microscopy has shown that a very thin continuous space exists between the alveolar cells and capillary endothelium and that this space is continuous with the interstitial connective tissue surrounding airways and larger blood vessels in the lungs. The osmotic pressure exerted by plasma proteins drains any fluid from the space so that the space is of negligible size. In the normal situation hydrostatic osmotic and tissue time pressures are nicely balanced (Fig. 19.1 a). Increase in capillary pressure may cause increased filtration and interstitial oedema which may initially be limited by lymphatic drainage. Further increase in filtration may lead to substantial oedema of the interstitial space. The interstitial oedema extends in the form of a cuff around small airways and blood vessels (Fig. 19.2). This produces important local changes in ventilation and perfusion:

1 Small airways become narrowed by interstitial oedema.
2 The lung tissue becomes firm and non-compliant—less air enters the zone on inspiration; during expiration closure of the airways occurs early leading to the production of rhonchi.
3 On inspiration when the airways eventually open they do so with a click—producing crepitations (p. 39).

4 Reduced ventilation of the firm non-compliant zone leads to local hypoxic and reflex arteriolar constriction and in addition the accumulated interstitial oedema may compress vessels resulting in reduced perfusion to the zone (blood is directed to less affected areas—an appropriate compensation).

5 Defective perfusion may lead to defective local production of surfactant.

6 Distortion of the cuffed bronchiolar/vascular bundles in the lung may cause irritation of vagal sensory endings ('J' receptors) leading to reflex stimulation of ventilation.

Because of the effect of gravity, capillary filtration is always greatest in the lower zones and interstitial oedema, cuffing, crepitations etc. are all more marked at the base of the lungs. Ventilation and perfusion become directed increasingly to the upper zones.

ALVEOLAR OEDEMA

Further increase in interstitial oedema which overloads the capacity of the lymphatics to preserve a state of balance may lead to alveolar oedema. The surface tension of the lung layer draws fluid into the alveoli (Fig. 19.1 c). In doing so the diameter of the alveolar bubble becomes reduced and surface tension increases. The effect of surface tension is to some extent counteracted by the surfactant layer but this may become defective with reduced blood flow. When imbalance becomes severe fluid may pour into the alveoli and accumulate in the airways. In florid pulmonary oedema pink fluid and foam are coughed up in large quantities.

Symptoms of pulmonary oedema

Shortness of breath is the principal symptom. This may be accompanied by:
exercise dyspnoea;
tachypnoea;
cough;
orthopnoea and paroxysmal nocturnal dyspnoea;
Cheyne Stokes Respiration;
finally extreme dyspnoea, cyanosis, coughing up of foaming sputum, haemoptysis.

Mild pulmonary oedema may cause no symptoms at rest but exercise dyspnoea is inevitable. More severe oedema causes breathlessness at rest and often an irritating cough.

ORTHOPNOEA

Typically orthopnoea is present (but also occurs in other forms of dyspnoea).

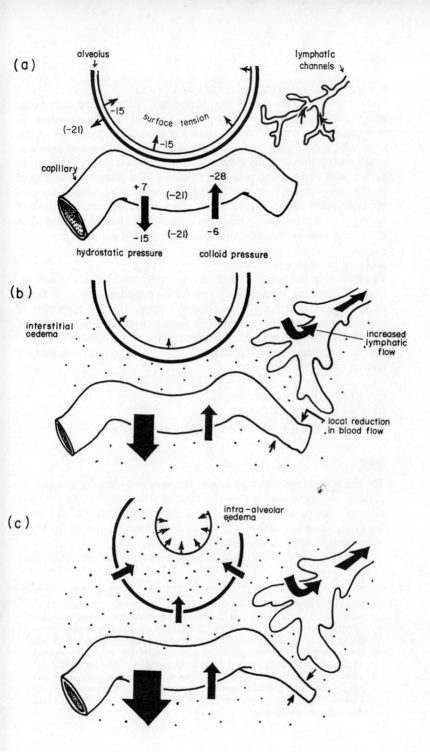

(a)

alveolus

lymphatic channels

−15

(−21)

surface tension

−15

capillary

+7

(−21)

−28

(−21)

(−21)

−15

−6

hydrostatic pressure

colloid pressure

(b)

interstitial oedema

increased lymphatic flow

local reduction in blood flow

(c)

intra−alveolar oedema

PAROXYSMAL NOCTURNAL DYSPNOEA (PND)

PND may occur—the patient characteristically wakes in the early hours with wheezy cough and severe dyspnoea. This episode may sometimes be indistinguishable from nocturnal attacks of bronchial asthma. One of the most helpful distinguishing features is the complaint of *morning* tightness, cough and dyspnoea by the asthmatic patient which is generally lacking in patient with PND due to pulmonary oedema. The precise mechanism of production of orthopnoea and PND is debatable and probably complex but one important factor may be the effect of gravity causing spread of basal pulmonary oedema to relatively oedema-free areas of the lung when the patient reclines, without important improvement in the bases.

CHEYNE STOKES RESPIRATION

This is waxing and waning ventilation generally with periods of apnoea. Cyclical breathing is commonly present in pulmonary oedema but is rarely sufficiently striking to be remarked upon. It is an expression of unstable ventilatory control due to a slowed circulation time, increased ventilatory drive and hypoxia. Fulminant pulmonary oedema is characterised by extreme respiratory distress with wheezing and commonly a rattling sound on breathing.

CYANOSIS AND THE COUGHING UP
OF FOAMY PINK SPUTUM

In this situation ventilation may be impeded and the P_{CO_2} may rise.

Signs

The character of the breathing may be laboured and wheezing or rapid and panting and sometimes with a fine rattling sound audible. In mild pulmonary oedema the only sign may be fine crepitations at the bases. Generally these are mainly mid or end-inspiratory in timing (p. 39). In some cases widespread fine rhonchi are audible.

There may be obvious signs of the cause of the oedema—particularly

---

Fig. 19.1. *Pulmonary oedema*
Diagram of an alveolus and pulmonary capillary. (a) *Normal situation*; approximate values for hydrostatic and colloid pressures in mmHg. These forces are in equilibrium or slightly in favour of fluid reabsorption so that the interstitial space is negligible at alveolar level. (b) *Pulmonary oedema*. Increase in pulmonary pressure leads to increased transudation of fluid. Increase in lymphatic fluid transport. At this stage interstitial oedema involves mainly the bronchovascular connective tissue (Fig. 19.2). (c) *Severe pulmonary oedema*. There is now separation of the fluid film from the alveolar surface and intra-alveolar oedema.

mitral or aortic valvular heart disease or cardiac enlargement with the characteristic sustained impulse of left ventricular enlargement. A third or fourth heart sound (or gallop) is a particularly valuable sign when the cause of the dyspnoea is in doubt.

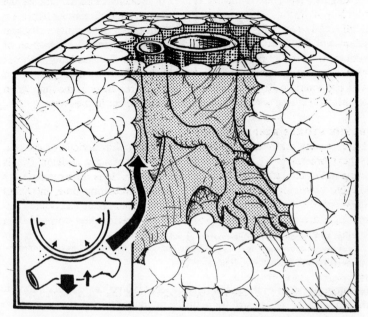

Fig. 19.2. Diagrammatic representation of the formation of interstitial oedema extending in the form of a 'cuff' around the bronchovascular bundle.

X-ray changes

The heart may be enlarged and pulmonary vessels may appear to be prominent, particularly those to the upper lobes. Mild pulmonary oedema may cause no radiological features. Kerley 'B' lines are very useful evidence of established pulmonary oedema (Fig. 19.3). These comprise short horizontal linear opacities which are found next to the pleural surfaces in the costo-phrenic angles. They are probably caused by dilated lymphatic channels in interlobular septa. Blotchy lung shadowing particularly near the hilum is common in severe pulmonary oedema. A fine mottling is occasionally seen in persistent pulmonary oedema.

Functional disturbance

Spirometry usually reveals a restrictive pattern of ventilatory impairment but prolonged expiratory time and reduced FEV_1/VC fraction are common. Hyperventilation is usual and the Pco_2 is low in all but the most severe cases. There is generally arterial hypoxia but this is often modest when the

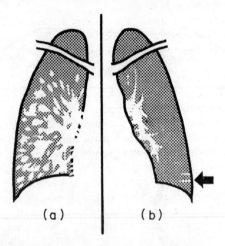

Fig. 19.3. *Radiographic appearances in pulmonary oedema*
(a) Severe pulmonary oedema. (b) Early pulmonary oedema. The arrow indicates the appearance of Kerley 'B' lines.

radiological extent of the pulmonary oedema is considered (a testimony to the efficiency of the redistribution of the pulmonary circulation away from oedematous underventilated areas).

Treatment

PRIMARY DISTURBANCE
Where pulmonary oedema results from valvular heart disease, renal failure, hypertension or other obvious primary disturbance, special measures will be required.

OXYGEN
Oxygen should be given in as high a concentration as practicable.

DIURETIC
Intravenous frusemide (40–80 mg) is generally very effective within a few hours. Sometimes improvement is dramatic and evident within 15 minutes before any notable increase in urine formation by the kidneys—an effect attributable to a peripheral effect of frusemide causing increased venous capacitance.

DIGITALISATION
This may be helpful when failing left ventricular function is important.

OPIATES
Morphia is particularly useful and opiates perhaps act by reducing fear and ventilatory drive and possibly also by inducing relaxation of sympathetically-mediated peripheral vasoconstriction.

EXCEPTIONAL MEASURES
Venous cuffs applied to the arms and legs may improve the situation for a short time in the critically ill patient.

α-adrenergic blocking agents have recently found a place in the management of serious pulmonary oedema particularly if it persists despite other measures. Phenoxybenzamine and phentolamine are the preparations most frequently employed. Administration is by carefully regulated continuous infusion. Peripheral vasodilatation is induced which improves the effectiveness of left ventricular emptying at the expense of some fall in blood pressure. Use of these agents requires continuous central venous pressure measurement and considerable expertise.

IPPV. In patients overwhelmed by fulminating pulmonary oedema intermittent positive pressure ventilation (IPPV) is occasionally lifesaving. The principal benefits which follow are:

1, improved clearing of foam and secretions by bronchial suction; 2, the ability to administer really high concentrations of oxygen continuously if necessary; and 3, the relief of exhaustion and terror by the use of powerful sedation. Some authorities support the use of high inflation pressures throughout the breathing cycle with the aim of 'pushing' fluid back into the pulmonary capillaries. Such measures can, however, cause embarrassment of the circulation as the increased airway pressure is transmitted directly to the pulmonary capillaries (and especially to those in the less oedematous areas).

CHAPTER 20 · PNEUMOTHORAX AND PLEURAL EFFUSION

PNEUMOTHORAX

Air may enter the pleural space from the lung or rarely from the outside as in the case of major chest trauma or thoracotomy. The intrapleural pressure is normally negative owing to the retractive force of lung elastic recoil (p. 8) so that once a communication is established between atmosphere and the pleural space the lung tends to deflate.

Spontaneous pneumothorax

The most common form of pneumothorax occurs spontaneously, usually in previously healthy young males. The source of the air leak is usually a tiny bleb on the surface of the lung near the apex.

The condition usually presents with the development of sudden unilateral pain which may be pleuritic and severe and accompanied by pallor, tachycardia and sweating. Breathlessness may follow if the pneumothorax is large or under tension (see below).

Physical signs

The principal physical sign is **diminution of breath sounds on the affected side**; in the absence of dullness to percussion this is usually most apparent anterio ly in the semirecumbent position. Hyperresonance is usually unimpressive. Small left-sided pneumothoraces may give rise to a sticky clicking sound in time with the heart.

The chest X-ray

The diagnosis is confirmed by chest X-ray. A fine crescentic line is found almost parallel to the chest wall outside which no lung markings are seen.

Tension pneumothorax

Tension pneumothorax constitutes something of a medical emergency. It arises in a small proportion of spontaneous pneumothoraces in which the communication between lung and pleural space acts as a valve permitting air to enter the pleural space during inspiration but closing during expiration. This results in more and more air accumulating in the pleural space which compresses the affected lung to about the size of a hand. The pressure within the pleural space may become positive throughout almost all the breathing cycle. The mediastinum becomes pushed to the opposite side and expansion of the opposite lung becomes impeded. The high mean thoracic pressure begins to impede return of blood to the heart and shock develops. Death may ensue from the combined effects of acute ventilatory and circulatory failure.

Signs

The signs of tension pneumothorax are increasing respiratory distress, tachypnoea and tachycardia and evidence of mediastinal shift as judged by movement of the trachea or cardiac apex.

Treatment

No treatment is required for very small pneumothoraces. There is no need to hospitalise such patients provided they are intelligent and able to return rapidly for attention if worsening symptoms develop. Pneumothoraces in which the lung is less than 2 cm from the chest wall resolve in about 2 weeks. Usually the pneumothorax occupies more than half of the chest and in this case active treatment is preferable as resolution is otherwise very protracted.

Tension pneumothorax demands immediate treatment. An intercostal catheter of rubber or plastic is introduced in the mid clavicular line in the 3rd interspace or in the axilla in the 4th or 5th interspace and connected to an underwater seal (Fig. 20.1). (Some clinicians favour the use of a rubber and plastic flutter valve which is equally satisfactory and permits the patient to be mobile.) Air bubbles out at each expiration or cough and, if the lung perforation has sealed, bubbles soon stop. The fluid level is then seen to swing with each breath from about -3 cm water to -10. If there is no further bubbling after 24 hours and the chest X-ray shows complete re-expansion of the lung the tube may be removed.

INDICATIONS FOR SURGICAL TREATMENT

In a few cases bubbling continues for 2–3 days. If it continues surgery is required to remove and oversew the lung perforation. About one in five spontaneous pneumothoraces recur, usually within the first year. If there are further recurrences or if an individual pneumothorax on the other side develops it is usual to recommend pleurodesis.

Pleurodesis

A pleural reaction is then generated with a view to producing fibrous obliteration of the pleural space. Some surgeons favour the use of talc and others favour stripping of part of the parietal pleura. Both methods give reliable security against subsequent pneumothorax.

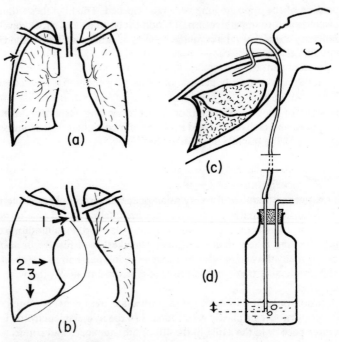

Fig. 20.1. *Pneumothorax*
(a) Radiographic appearances of a small right pneumothorax.
(b) Radiographic appearances of a large tension pneumothorax on the right. 1. The trachea and mediastinum are displaced to the left. 2. The right lung has collapsed completely. 3. The diaphragm is depressed.
(c) Intercostal tube in place.
(d) Under-water seal. The end of the tube is 2–3 cm below the level of the water in the bottle. If intrapleural pressure rises above 2–3 cm H_2O air will bubble out. If intrapleural pressure becomes negative water rises up the tube only to fall again when intrapleural pressure falls towards atmospheric. The system operates as a simple one-way valve. When the pneumothorax has resolved the water level will generally be slightly negative throughout the respiratory cycle reflecting the normal fluctuations in intrapleural pressure and when the patient coughs air will no longer bubble out.

Pneumothorax accompanying other lung disease

In the older age group pneumothorax most often results from rupture of an emphysematous bulla in an individual with established chronic airways obstruction. In this situation an already disabled patient may be rendered critically ill by a relatively small pneumothorax. Treatment by intercostal drainage is generally satisfactory but a greater proportion continue to leak air for many days and eventually come to require thoracotomy and excision of the bullae.

A pneumothorax may result from rupture of lung cysts associated with advanced fibrosing alveolitis, other forms of lung fibrosis, eosinophilic granuloma etc. A lung abscess or carcinoma may break down and lead to the development of a bronchopleural fistula. In this situation a pyo-pneumothorax is generally present and this is a well-established persistent communication with the bronchial tree. Surgical treatment is always necessary.

PLEURAL EFFUSION

The discovery of pleural fluid is always important and demands explanation. Pleural effusion may complicate a wide variety of pulmonary conditions but discussion will be limited here to pleural effusion apparently occurring in isolation.

Signs

Factors indicating pleural effusion are outlined on p. 42.

Radiological features

Features apparent in radiology are outlined on p. 65.

Pleural aspiration

Useful information relating to the cause of the effusion can be obtained from pleural aspiration. Heavily bloodstained fluid suggests pulmonary malignancy unless there is strong suspicion of pulmonary embolism and infarction. Pleural effusions fall into two main groups: transudates which as a rule accompany generalised oedematous states and exudates which are derived from inflammation of the pleural membrane and adjacent tissues. It is not possible to discriminate between these groups completely but fluid with a high protein content (above about half of the serum protein value) is likely to be an exudate.

A pleural fluid lactic dehydrogenase (LDH) level of greater than 200 I.U. or more than 60 per cent of the serum LDH level is also characteristic of an exudate.

Cytological examination of the fluid is valuable if expertise is locally available. The patient should be tipped into various positions immediately before aspiration because cells tend to sediment into the dependent part of the pleural space and may not be sampled on aspiration. A large volume of fluid should be obtained and centrifuged and a smear of the sediment examined.

Bacteriological examination is important in the presence of fever after pneumonia or in suspected tuberculosis.

Pleural biopsy. A pleural biopsy should be performed whenever a diagnostic pleural aspiration is undertaken (Fig. 17.3). This technique is particularly effective in the diagnosis of tuberculous and malignant pleural effusions.

Pleural exudates

These are most commonly due to pulmonary malignant disease or infection. Pulmonary tuberculosis may cause pleural effusion in the early postprimary phase (p. 89) but this presentation of tuberculosis is now rather rare. The effusion is generally large, has a high protein content and contains mainly lymphocytes. Pleural effusion may develop after almost any form of bacterial or viral pneumonia but is not usually massive. The cells may be largely either polymorphs or lymphocytes and the fluid is usually extensive. Persistent recurrence of effusion suggests that a neoplasm may have been the cause of the original pneumonia. Acute pancreatitis may be associated with a left-sided effusion. The fluid contains a high level of amylase and the effusion may be in fistulous communication with a pancreatic pseudocyst.

Pleural transudates

Pleural effusions are common in florid right heart failure and in constrictive pericarditis. They may less commonly accompany other generalised oedematous states—for example renal failure or hypoproteinaemic states such as nephrotic syndrome or chronic hepatic failure. Right-sided pleural effusion may sometimes be due to ascitic fluid which may pass through congenital transdiaphragmatic communications on the right side. An ovarian fibroma may cause such a combination of ascites and pleural effusion (Meig's syndrome). Peritoneal dialysis fluid may produce a right-sided pleural effusion.

Pleural effusion is not uncommon amongst patients with rheumatoid arthritis. The effusion is usually small and sometimes asymptomatic. It usually resolves after some months. The diagnosis rests on clinical features of R.A. and on positive rheumatoid factor. Pleuritic pain and sometimes pleural effusion is one of the commoner features of systemic lupus erythematosus (SLE) in relapse. There may occasionally be underlying irregular lung infiltrations evident on the chest X-ray at this time. The diagnosis rests on other characteristic features of SLE, particularly skin rashes and arthritis, and on the finding of antinuclear factor and LE cells in the blood.

Treatment

The management of pleural effusion naturally depends upon treatment of the primary cause. Malignant pleural effusion may be very distressing and demoralising and there is some merit in weekly aspiration and instillation of nitrogen mustard as reaccumulation can generally be slowed and sometimes arrested by this means.

Empyema

This term signifies the presence of pus in the pleural cavity. Usually it arises after severe pneumonia, rupture of a lung abscess or after thoracic surgery. Rupture of the oesophagus may lead to a left-sided empyema particularly when it is due to invasion by a malignant tumour. Actinomycosis is a rare cause of empyema. Sometimes it progresses to form a discharging chest wall sinus.

The patient generally has a high swinging fever and is profoundly ill with a high leucocytosis. The collection of fluid is often loculated and difficult to aspirate. The radiological appearances may vary from the usual appearance of an effusion because of fibrous adhesions and loculation.

The management of empyema depends upon antibiotic treatment and attention to the primary cause. Sometimes decortication (operative stripping of the pleura and pus-filled cavities) is necessary.

Haemothorax

Bleeding into the pleural cavity may complicate
a Chest injury—especially with rib fracture
b Rupture of pleural adhesions
c Pulmonary infarction (usually not massive)
d Anticoagulant therapy especially with a or b.
If massive intrapleural bleeding occurs and the patient becomes shocked, blood transfusion and even emergency surgical exploration to arrest bleeding may occasionally be required.

If repeated aspiration fails to remove the blood clot a fibrinous rind may develop which may become organised, lead to fibrosis and cause permanently restricted movement of the chest. In this situation a thoracotomy may be required for removal of the fibrinous rind.

Chylothorax

A rare phenomenon characterised by the accumulation of lymph in the pleural cavity. It is caused by leakage from the thoracic duct or other major lymphatic channel as a consequence of surgical trauma, other injury or malignant invasion. The chylous effusion reaccumulates rapidly after aspiration. Repeated aspiration leads to protein and lymphocyte depletion. Surgical treatment is required if it persists. Tying of the thoracic duct is generally effective.

Dry pleurisy

Pleurisy is a term used merely to indicate inflammation of the pleura and the characteristic pain that this causes. Any of the conditions which give rise to an exudative pleural effusion may cause dry pleurisy.

BORNHOLM DISEASE
(Epidemic myalgia)

This uncommon condition is characterised by extremely severe immobilising pleuritic chest pain and sometimes abdominal pain with variable symptoms of fever and sometimes sore throat. The condition persists for several days before spontaneously resolving. It is due to infection with Coxackie B virus and the diagnosis may be confirmed by isolation of the virus from the throat or stool or retrospectively by observing a rising titre of specific antibody in the serum.

CHAPTER 21 · TRAUMA AND
THE LUNGS

Penetrating wounds of the chest

Stabbing and similar penetrating injuries commonly cause a pneumothorax from lung perforation or sucking wound and may also result in
intrathoracic haemorrhage. The management comprises infusion of blood
and plasma, drainage of the pneumothorax and if there is evidence of
continued bleeding emergency thoracotomy. Gaping sucking wounds of
the chest may rapidly cause ventilatory failure.

Rib fracture

Fracture of ribs is usually due to a fall or direct trauma to the chest but in
muscular patients with severe airways obstruction and those with osteoporosis ribs may be fractured by strenuous coughing. The cardinal sign is
exquisite local tenderness. Distressing pain may lead to suppression of
coughing and retention of bronchial secretions with subsequent pneumonia.
Pain causes splinting of the affected side and progressive lung collapse may
occur due to failure to take occasional deeper breaths. Rib fracture is a
serious event in the elderly. A combination of adequate analgesia (sometimes with the help of intercostal block), antibiotic therapy and encouragement to cough and take occasional deep breaths may be all that is required
but occasionally tracheostomy with or without IPPV is necessary. Pneumothorax and haemothorax may complicate the fracture.

Multiple rib fractures—flail chest

Massive blunt injury to the chest occurs in car crashes and some industrial
accidents and constitutes an immediate emergency. If more than two or
three ribs are fractured in two places a substantial segment of the chest
wall loses its rigidity and may flap in and out during breathing—this
results in very inefficient ventilation and may be enough to cause acute
respiratory failure with hypercapnia and hypoxia. IPPV is essential in this
situation and, as it is required for a few weeks to ensure splinting of the
chest whilst the ribs unite, it is usual to perform an elective tracheostomy
at an early stage. In the early hours or days heavy sedation and curarisation
may be necessary to prevent respiratory distress and excessive displacement of the fractured ribs.

Crush injury to the lung

Blunt crushing injuries to the chest, with or without rib fractures, can cause profound pulmonary disturbance over the course of the first few days after injury. Widespread fluffy shadowing on the chest X-ray reflects alveolar haemorrhage and oedema and there is progressive dyspnoea and cyanosis. This sometimes proves fatal despite IPPV and oxygen.

Shock lung

This is a term which has grown into use to describe diffuse parenchymal alveolar haemorrhage, consolidation and oedema accompanying trauma and states of profound shock. It is of delayed onset usually appearing 1 to 3 days after the episode of shock or trauma. The first signs are tachypnoea, hyperventilation and crepitations which progress. Cyanosis usually follows and this may be resistant to oxygen administration. It seems particularly likely to occur when there is extensive muscle necrosis associated with the trauma and some workers feel that embolisation of clot and metabolites from necrotic tissue may be important in its causation. Others feel that a period of pulmonary under-perfusion is the critical predisposing factor. Severely ill patients in this situation are subject to many pulmonary hazards: inhalation of vomit and secretions, fat embolism, thromboembolism, pneumonia, septicaemia, oxygen toxicity and pulmonary oedema from infusion of blood, plasma and electrolyte solutions so that it is possible that there is no single mechanism of causation.

Management centres upon ensuring adequate oxygenation usually with controlled IPPV. Cortiscosteroids and heparin (where appropriate) may be helpful; there is a high mortality.

CHAPTER 22 · OCCUPATIONAL LUNG DISEASE

The term pneumoconiosis is reserved for a group of occupational lung diseases characterised by a parenchymal reaction (which is usually fibrosis) to inhaled mineral dust. Although this group is the best-known form of occupational lung disease a variety of other reactions to dusts, gases, fumes and vapours are encountered. The character of the lung reaction depends upon the chemical nature of the substance, its physical form and the intensity and duration of exposure and it may also be influenced by the presence of pre-existing lung disease. The clinical features of occupational lung disease are in the main non-specific and the diagnosis depends to a large extent on obtaining a comprehensive occupational history.

Penetration, deposition and clearance of particles within the lung

The distance to which inhaled particles penetrate the respiratory tract depends principally upon their size. The nose is a surprisingly effective 'filter' and extracts almost all particles with a diameter greater than about 20μ as well as a large proportion of particles which are smaller than this. Particles between 3 and 9μ in diameter which are not deposited in the nose tend mainly to be deposited in the bronchial tree proximal to the respiratory bronchiole. They may then be removed by ciliary action within 12 hours or so. Particles smaller than 3μ are most likely to penetrate as far as the alveoli and those of the order of 1μ are most likely to be deposited there. Clearance of these particles is effected by alveolar macrophages. These cells are phagocytic and mobile; they engulf deposited particles and transport them to the terminal bronchiole from which they are carried on the 'mucociliary escalator' eventually to be swallowed or expectorated in the sputum. Some particles are toxic to macrophages in which case transport to the terminal bronchiole is impaired. The particles tend to be liberated and re-engulfed repeatedly by macrophages and particles may accumulate in respiratory bronchioles. A proportion gain entry to the interstitial tissue of the lung and may ultimately be transported proximally via lymphatic channels. (See Fig. 22.1.)

Bronchial reactions

Acute tracheitis and bronchitis

These reactions are most likely to arise following rare accidental exposure

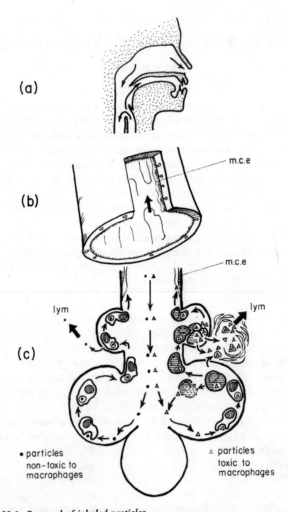

(a)

(b)

m.c.e

m.c.e

lym

lym

(c)

• particles
non-toxic to
macrophages

△ particles
toxic to
macrophages

Fig. 22.1. *Removal of inhaled particles*
The arrows indicate the routes for disposal of inhaled particles (a) in the upper
respiratory tract, (b) in the bronchi and (c) within the lobule.
(c) particles deposited in alveoli are ingested by phagocytic macrophages which
migrate towards the terminal bronchiole. Most non-toxic particles (shown
at the left) are successfully transported to the mucociliary escalator (m.c.e.).
Some penetrate the alveolar wall if the inhaled load is heavy and are carried
away by the lymphatics (lym). Particles (such as silica) which are toxic to macrophages may be liberated after death of the macrophage and be subsequently
re-ingested. The particles may become covered with a proteinaceous coating.
Damaged macrophages and particles tend to accumulate particularly in respiratory bronchioles. Coated particles which penetrate the alveolar walls
appear to be capable of exciting a fibrous reaction.

to irritant fumes or gases or aerosols of irritant liquids (especially ammonia, chlorine).

Occupational asthma

A number of occupations involve exposure to allergenic organic dusts. Atopic individuals are particularly likely to develop hypersensitivity which may express itself as asthma. Particularly heavy exposure may result in the sensitisation even of non-atopic individuals. Amongst the best-known examples are asthma occurring in: 1, flour-mill workers due to sensitivity to the wheat-weevil (*Sitophilus granarius*) and other contaminants of stored grain; 2, woodworkers due to sensitivity to some redwood and hardwood dusts; 3, printers due to sensitivity to gum acacia in some printers' inks; 4, workers handling fur and feathers due to sensitisation to the dusts. Asthmatic reactions may be immediate or delayed and sometimes both reactions occur.

Toluene di-isocyanate (TDI) is an important special case. TDI is used in the manufacture of polyurethane products, particularly foams, and workers exposed to it may develop asthmatic reactions. A proportion of these individuals may develop extreme sensitivity to the substance so that even trivial exposure to it may provoke severe symptoms which sometimes persist for several days.

Byssinosis

This disorder occurs in cotton workers employed in the card room after many years of heavy exposure to cotton dust. It is characterised by tightness in the chest and cough occurring promptly on entering the mill particularly after a few days' absence. The symptoms are particularly likely to develop in individuals who already have chronic bronchitis or asthma. There is no parenchymal lung involvement and no abnormalities are evident on the chest X-ray. There is some evidence to suggest that both Type I and Type III reactions may occur in the bronchi in response to an antigenic fraction of cotton dust.

Alveolar reactions

Extrinsic allergic alveolitis (see p. 137)

Most varieties of extrinsic allergic alveolitis arise as a consequence of heavy occupational exposure to allergenic dusts, e.g. Farmer's lung.

Pulmonary oedema

Acute pulmonary oedema may occur following inhalation of some toxic gases including sulphur dioxide, chlorine and ammonia. The reaction may be prompt or delayed.

Welding yields a variety of oxides of nitrogen and, if it is undertaken in very confined spaces, exposure to the gases may result in the development of acute pulmonary oedema with cough, tightness, dyspnoea, widespread crepitations and radiological shadowing. This may resolve slowly and re-appear later, sometimes after an interval of some weeks. Fresh silage yields nitrogen dioxide and workers entering silo towers may develop similar pulmonary oedema which may be delayed in appearance.

Metal fume may cause pulmonary irritation and pulmonary oedema or pneumonia. Cadmium workers may develop severe reactions with subse-quent lung destruction. Lesser reactions follow exposure to magnesium, vanadium, zinc and tungsten fume. 'Metal fume fever' is a term used to describe generalised symptoms of malaise which may accompany exposure.

Pneumoconiosis

Coal-worker's pneumoconiosis

There are about 40,000 persons in the U.K. at the present time with established coal-worker's pneumoconiosis. The development of pneumo-coniosis is directly related to the total exposure to dust which is deter-mined by the particular working conditions experienced by the individual. Dust exposure varies in different parts of the coal mine and is heaviest at the coal-face. Strenuous efforts have been made to reduce dust exposure during the last 20 years and there has been some reduction in the incidence of new cases. There is an important distinction to be made between the two major categories of coal-worker's pneumoconiosis.

SIMPLE PNEUMOCONIOSIS

This term refers to the accumulation within the lung tissue of relatively small (up to 5 mm in diameter) aggregations of coal particles which are fairly uniformly dispersed and evident on the chest X-ray as a delicate micronodular mottling. A series of X-rays is published by the International Labour Office which allows standardised categorisation of the radiological appearances. Numerals (0, 1, 2, 3, 4) are used to indicate the profusion of opacities and letters to indicate size (p, q, r for rounded opacities and s, t, u for irregular opacities). Examination of the lungs may show localised dilatation of the air spaces immediately adjacent to the aggregations of coal (sometimes referred to as focal emphysema). **Simple pneumoconiosis causes no important symptoms, signs or physiological impairment.** There is to date no strong evidence that its presence influences subsequent health or life expectancy. The benign nature of simple pneumoconiosis is sometimes not appreciated and there is a widespread tendency to attribute almost any respiratory symptoms to pneumoconiosis once simple pneumoconiosis has been recognised from the chest X-ray. An alternative explanation—usually in the shape of chronic bronchitis, asthma or heart disease—should always be suspected in such individuals.

PROGRESSIVE MASSIVE FIBROSIS (PMF)

In PMF larger opacities are evident on the chest X-ray. The ILO classifications A, B and C are used to indicate opacities of greater than 1 cm in diameter.

A   Sum of diameters of opacities less than 5 cm.
B   Sum of diameters of opacities more than 5 cm but the opacities occupy less than one-third of the area of the right lung field.
C   Greater than B.

Category C is more commonly accompanied by symptoms of breathlessness and detectable physiological impairment in the form of a restrictive ventilatory defect and a variable reduction in transfer factor. On the other hand extensive PMF may be present without notable symptoms or important physiological impairment. Categories B and C do carry a higher than expected risk of subsequent respiratory illness and premature death.

The lungs contain condensed masses of fibrous tissue heavily infiltrated with collections of coal dust particles. Sometimes the centres of these masses become softened and they rupture into the lung tissue. Large amounts of black material may be coughed up and part of the radiological shadowing may be found to have disappeared.

It is not clear why some coal workers develop PMF whilst others equally exposed to coal dust do not. The condition is not closely related to the silica content of the workings or to pulmonary tuberculosis and it may perhaps depend on obscure individual differences in reticuloendothelial function.

CAPLAN'S SYNDROME (RHEUMATOID COAL PNEUMOCONIOSIS)

Coal workers with rheumatoid arthritis may develop multiple nodular pulmonary opacities, usually about 0·5 to 2 cm in diameter, which may superficially resemble PMF. Usually, however, the nodules are accompanied by only very modest evidence of simple pneumoconiosis and there may be no background stippling at all. Sometimes the manifestations of rheumatoid arthritis are very slight or even absent but rheumatoid factor is always present in the serum. The radiological appearances may sometimes be misinterpreted as being due to multiple pulmonary metastases.

Silicosis

Silicosis is now relatively uncommon because of the widespread recognition of the hazards of respirable silicaceous dust. There is still a risk of harmful exposure in certain quarrying, mining and sandblasting operations. Foundry workers are exposed to silica dust from the sand used in forming moulds. Sand particles become partly fused and adherent to the castings and removal of this material (fettling and blasting) is hazardous. Workers involved in maintaining the refactory lining of kilns and furnaces are also at risk as are workers in the ceramic industry involved in dry milling of ingredients or dry finishing of fired articles.

Clinical features

Simple nodular silicosis, like simple coal-worker's pneumoconiosis, is not usually accompanied by symptoms and may be apparent only from the chest X-ray appearances. With advance of the disease a troublesome cough tends to develop. Advanced nodular silicosis with widespread confluent radiological shadowing or large masses and streaky lung fibrosis is accompanied by increasing breathlessness, a restrictive ventilatory defect and impairment of gas transfer. Another form of silicosis takes the form of a diffuse interstitial fibrosis. Occasionally after relatively short but heavy exposure to silical dust the disease may progress rapidly resulting in widespread fibrosis and honeycomb change within a matter of months (acute silicosis). Silicosis shows a general tendency to progress long after removal from exposure. Silicosis seems to predispose to pulmonary tuberculosis and leads to a particularly vicious fibrous reaction to the infection.

Pathological features

Microscopic examination of silicotic nodules shows them to be composed of concentric whorls of densely arranged collagen fibres showing varying amounts of hyaline change. Silica particles may be found in these nodules and also within macrophages and within the alveoli where there may be proliferation of adjacent cells. The most proximal alveoli opening off respiratory bronchioles seem to be most heavily involved.

Siderosis

Dust containing iron and its oxides is encountered in haematite mines, at various stages in the iron and steel industry and in welding. It gives rise to a simple pneumoconiosis (siderosis) which produces a striking mottled appearance on the chest X-ray because of high radiodensity of iron but which is not accompanied by symptoms, signs or physiological defect. Other metals such as antimony and tin may produce a similar picture.

Asbestos

Asbestos is a collective term which refers to a number of naturally occurring fibrous mineral silicates which have found widespread use throughout the civilised world on account of their ability to bind other materials together and because of striking resistance to heat and corrosive agents. The most important forms of asbestos are:

1. *Chrysotile (white asbestos)*

This is a 'serpentine' form of asbestos; the fibres are wispy, flexible and often relatively long. Chrysotile accounts for most of the asbestos used. It appears as a bonding agent in asbestos-cement products—pipes, tiles, roofing materials etc.—and is also included in asbestos-paper insulating materials and brake-linings.

2. *The amphibole group*

These forms have straighter more brittle fibres. Crocidolite (blue asbestos), amosite and anthophyllite are the most important members of the group. Longer fibres can be carded, spun and made into heat-resistant fabric; shorter fibres tend to be used in other forms of insulation and a filler and reinforcing agents in a variety of plastic, rubber and paint products. Despite its universal presence the great bulk of asbestos is safely bound within composite materials and important exposure is still largely confined to certain occupations in which actual dust is produced. Amongst those at risk are pipe laggers and industrial plumbers who come into contact with asbestos insulation and workers in the construction industries who process asbestos-cement products, laminated asbestos materials used in fireproof partitions and sprayed wall coverings. In some industries (e.g. shipbuilding) heavy environmental contamination may result in exposure of other workers.

Consequences of heavy exposure

I. ASBESTOSIS

Heavy industrial exposure to asbestos dust may lead to slowly progressive diffuse pulmonary fibrosis. This may be evident on the chest X-ray as a fine basal haziness or mottling sometimes accompanied by streaky shadows. Clinically the disease presents with cough and slowly progressive dyspnoea which may later be accompanied by cyanosis and clubbing. The earliest clinical sign is usually fine basal crepitations. Tests of pulmonary function reveal reduction in vital capacity and lung compliance and a progressive impairment of gas transfer. The condition may progress even after exposure has ceased.

2. BRONCHIAL CARCINOMA

A high proportion of individuals with established pulmonary asbestosis die from bronchial carcinoma. Carcinoma occurring in this situation qualifies for compensation under the Industrial Injuries Acts.

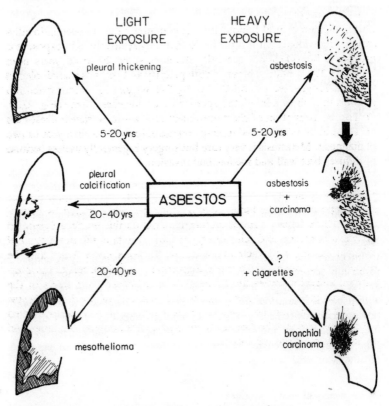

Fig. 22.2. *Pulmonary diseases relating to exposure to asbestos*

There appears to be an increased incidence of bronchial carcinoma amongst those exposed to asbestos but without asbestosis. Cigarette smoking and asbestos may exert a synergistic effect in its causation.

Consequences of even trivial exposure

I. PLEURAL THICKENING AND PLEURAL CALCIFICATION

Areas of pleural thickening and calcified pleural plaques are very common in workers exposed to asbestos and are also found amongst members of their families and those who have had quite trivial exposure. The plaques are visible on the chest X-ray but are quite harmless. They serve as a 'marker' of asbestos exposure and may develop many years later.

2. MESOTHELIOMA

This malignant pleural tumour is most commonly seen in occupationally-exposed individuals but it is probable that only relatively light exposure is necessary. Mesothelioma generally develops some 20 to 40 years after exposure. The condition presents with pleurisy and perhaps a small pleural effusion. Progressive pleural thickening follows due to tumour extension and this may show a lobulated appearance on the chest X-ray (Fig. 22.2). Progressive restriction of chest movement and severe persistent chest pain are features of the advanced disease and death follows within a year or two of diagnosis. Metastasis is very rare but surgery is generally useless because of diffuse chest wall and mediastinal invasion.

3. ASBESTOS BODIES

After deposition in the lungs asbestos fibres become engulfed by macrophages which deposit a proteinaceous material on their surface. Repeated ingestion liberation and reingestion probably results in the production of asbestos bodies with their characteristic bulbous ends. They may be present in the sputum and a small proportion may gain access to the interstitium. Asbestos bodies are thought to be produced from fibres of the amphibole group. They serve as another 'marker' of previous asbestos exposure but they are not essential to the diagnosis of the asbestos-related conditions. Asbestos bodies are found fairly commonly in the lungs and sputum in industrialised societies.

CHAPTER 23 · HYPOXIA AND OXYGEN THERAPY

Hypoxia

Hypoxia is ultimately a cellular phenomenon. Mitochondrial activity continues by aerobic metabolism until very low intracellular oxygen tensions are reached (of the order of 0·15 kPa or about 1 mmHg Po_2) after which anaerobic metabolism appears. This is inefficient and leads to accumulation of lactic acid which is a by-product.

Tissues vary greatly in their susceptibility to hypoxia. Broadly those tissues with a high extraction rate are the most susceptible (brain, heart). Hypoxia becomes important when:

1 It causes reduction in function of the organ with remote adverse effects which could themselves worsen hypoxia (the positive-feedback situation).

2 It threatens to cause irreversible damage to the organ.

It is often difficult to estimate when these two situations exist. The diagnosis of hypoxia relies heavily on the overall assessment of the factors known to be important in determining the rate of oxygen delivery to the tissues. These factors are summarised in Fig. 23.1.

1. Arterial oxygen content

This is determined by

a Haemoglobin concentration.

b Factors affecting the shape of the dissociation curve such as pH and Pco_2.

c Ventilation/perfusion relationships within the lung. When these include an important shunt component the mixed venous oxygen content influences arterial oxygen content and venous content is itself determined by oxygen delivery to the tissues.

2. Cardiac output

Oxygen delivery to the body (or oxygen flux) is determined by:

$$\text{Arterial oxygen content} \times \text{Cardiac output}$$

Circulatory impairment is potentially a much more potent cause of hypoxia than pulmonary impairment.

3. Distribution

Local vasoconstriction or vasodilatation is determined by reflex and local metabolic factors which can have a marked effect on oxygen delivery. The effect can be in the direction of aggravating hypoxia or ameliorating it (for example hypercapnia, hypoxia and hypotension all have a vasodilator effect in the cerebral circulation).

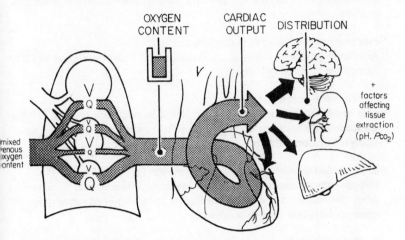

Fig. 23.1. Factors which require to be considered in the assessment of hypoxia.

4. Other factors

Other factors which are of some importance include those affecting tissue oxygen extraction. Increase in H^+, P_{CO_2} and temperature all shift the oxygen dissociation curve to the right and facilitate the unloading of oxygen.

From the foregoing discussion it should be evident that:
1 **The arterial oxygen content is only one factor which determines the development and severity of hypoxia.**
2 **The only part of the oxygen delivery system which can readily be influenced by oxygen administration is the arterial oxygen content.**

Oxygen therapy

Indications

The indications for oxygen therapy are difficult to define rigidly. Broadly speaking oxygen should be given when arterial hypoxaemia is an important threat to the patient's security provided that it is safe to do so.

Limiting factors

The two main considerations limiting the use of oxygen are:
1 The danger of inducing hypoventilation in patients with poor respiratory drive who may be relying on the ventilatory stimulus of hypoxia.
2 The danger of oxygen toxicity with the administration of high concentrations.

CORRECTION OF ARTERIAL HYPOXAEMIA

Arterial hypoxaemia arises as a consequence of underventilation of all or part of the circulating blood.

1. *Alveolar hypoventilation*

This results in hypoxaemia and reciprocal hypercapnia (p. 16). Oxygen administration may completely reverse the hypoxaemia. The problem of underventilation remains.

2. *Disturbed ventilation/perfusion relationships* (p. 20)

Oxygen administration may completely reverse the arterial hypoxaemia from this cause as the blood perfusing underventilated areas then encounters adequate oxygen tensions.

3. *Right–left shunts*

Such shunts may be regarded as an extreme form of 2 except that the blood passing to the shunt is inaccessible to the increased oxygen tension. A small amount of oxygen can be carried in the plasma of the blood traversing the lungs—about 2 ml per 100 ml for every 101 kPa (760 mmHg) partial pressure of oxygen—and this can be useful in the critically placed patient.

Other indications

Oxygen administration is desirable in situations where the cardiac output is seriously low even if arterial oxygen saturation is normal. A high concentration may increase the oxygen content of blood slightly by virtue of plasma solubility. Very severe anaemia and carbon monoxide poisoning constitute further indications for oxygen administration.

Method of administration

ONE HUNDRED PER CENT OXYGEN

Most of the masks in general use, although supplied by 100 per cent oxygen, in fact achieve much lower inspired concentrations. An inspired through non-return valves and in the clinical situation this only occurs in the context of artificial ventilation. One hundred per cent oxygen may be indicated in exceptional circumstances; prolonged use is attended by the risk of oxygen toxicity.

MASKS DELIVERING 40–60 PER CENT

A variety of masks achieve inspired levels of this order and two are shown in Fig. 23.2. The actual inspired concentration depends upon a number of factors which include: rate of oxygen flow, breathing pattern (tidal volume, frequency and inspiratory flow rate) and the amount of rebreathing permitted by the mask. The effective concentration of oxygen is also influenced by the position of the mask on the face.

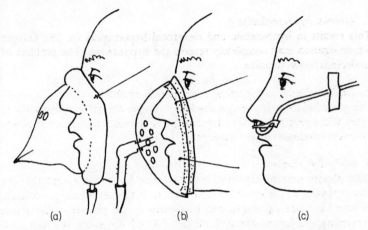

(a)   (b)   (c)

Fig. 23.2. *Oxygen administration—high concentration.* For patients with good ventilatory drive.
(a) Pneumask; (b) MC mask (Henleys Medical Supplies Ltd). These masks can deliver the equivalent of an inspired concentration of 40 to 60 per cent depending on oxygen flow rate and a number of other factors. (c) Nasal catheters. A short catheter is situated in each nostril penetrating only as far as the anterior nares.

Application

Masks in this group are appropriate in patients with good respiratory drive—severe asthma, infiltrative lung disorders, pneumonia, pulmonary oedema etc.

MASKS DELIVERING LOW OXYGEN
CONCENTRATIONS

These masks produce a fast-flowing stream of fixed low oxygen concentration (Fig. 23.3). In masks of this type air is entrained by a jet of oxygen. The inspired oxygen concentration is independent of breathing pattern, no rebreathing occurs and the position of the mask is less critical than is the case with some other masks. The concentration delivered is also relatively independent of the oxygen flow-rate, being determined by the geometry of the air-entrainment mechanism. A selection of masks giving 24, 28, and 35 per cent oxygen is available. In general these masks are well tolerated; some patients appreciate the breeze they produce but others are distressed by the noise.

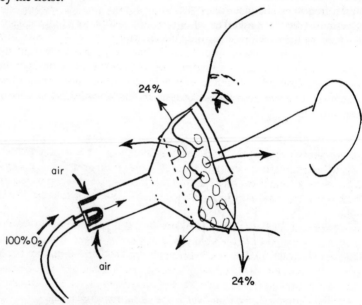

Fig. 23.3. *Oxygen administration—controlled low concentration*
Ventimask (Vickers Ltd).
Suitable for patients with impaired ventilatory drive. Unsuitable for patients with arterial hypoxaemia in other situations. A low concentration of oxygen is produced by the oxygen-driven air-entraining venturi and a high flow rate is maintained through the mask so that no room air or exhaled air is inspired. Note that masks are available which produce other higher concentrations (24 per cent, 28 per cent and 35 per cent in this range).

Application
Masks in this group may be indicated when severe hypoxia complicates an exacerbation of chronic bronchitis with established ventilatory failure (but see p. 170).

Note. Although these masks limit the extent of hypoventilation which may accompany oxygen administration they do not prevent it altogether.

Even 24 per cent oxygen increases the inspired Po_2 by about 2·8 kPa (21 mmHg) so that, if a patient was heavily dependent upon the hypoxic drive, the alveolar Pco_2 could theoretically rise by 2·3–2·8 kPa (17–21 mmHg) as he reduced ventilation until the arterial Po_2 reached its former level. In the case of a mask delivering 28 per cent the Pco_2 could conceivably rise by 5 or 6 kPa (say 40 to 50 mmHg).

NASAL OXYGEN ADMINISTRATION
Some patients do not tolerate covering of the face with a mask. Nasal administration overcomes this difficulty and also permits feeding and expectoration without interruption. Oxygen can be delivered by means of two short catheters which enter only the anterior nares or by means of a longer soft catheter reaching to the nasopharynx. Inspired levels of the order of 40 per cent may be obtained. Some patients breathe through the mouth but nasal administration even with the short catheters is often surprisingly effective nevertheless. Oxygen should be humidified to prevent nasal crusting.

OTHER METHODS
Oxygen tents provide an oxygen-rich environment but it is extremely difficult to maintain a constant inspired oxygen concentration. Oxygen tents severely limit ease of access to the patient for nursing purposes. Their main application is in childhood; children do not tolerate masks well.

A head-tent (Vickers Ltd) is occasionally useful in patients who require a low concentration of oxygen but are intolerant of masks. It comprises a transparent plastic curtain which surrounds the head and shoulders but is open at the bottom. A high flow of low oxygen concentration is directed downwards through the tent by means of an oxygen-driven air-entraining venturi housed in a dome from which the curtain is suspended.

**Oxygen therapy in exacerbations
of chronic bronchitis** (p. 170)

Domiciliary oxygen therapy (p. 231)

Hazards of oxygen therapy

1. HYPOVENTILATION (see above)

2. WITHDRAWAL OF OXYGEN
If oxygen is being given to a patient with severe hypoventilation it may be dangerous to withdraw it.

The dotted line in Fig. 2.6 shows the relationship between alveolar

Po_2 and Pco_2 when breathing air. The extent to which hypoventilation can progress is limited by hypoxia. For example if the Pco_2 rises to 12 kPa (90 mmHg) the Po_2 falls to about 4·7 kPa (35 mmHg). Survival is unusual if the arterial Po_2 falls much below 25 mmHg. When oxygen is administered much more severe hypoventilation can be tolerated. If oxygen is then withdrawn the patient will be plunged into catastrophic hypoxia. Even if ventilation is then increased, the body reserves of accumulated CO_2 will ensure that the alveolar Pco_2 remains elevated for some time.

If oxygen is being administered to a patient with severe hypoventilation of whatever cause, it must be administered **continuously** until ventilation has been improved.

3. RETROLENTAL FIBROPLASIA
Administration of high concentrations of oxygen (sufficient to produce an arterial Po_2 of over 19 kPa or approximately 140 mmHg) may produce retrolental fibroplasia in the neonatal period leading subsequently to variable degrees of blindness.

4. PULMONARY OXYGEN TOXICITY
High concentrations of oxygen cause damage to the alveoli. The earliest changes are those of capillary proliferation followed by intra-alveolar haemorrhage and exudation and the formation of hyaline membranes. Areas of collapse develop, lung compliance falls and gas transfer becomes progressively impaired leading ultimately to arterial hypoxaemia despite the high inspired concentration. Inhalation of 100 per cent oxygen causes reversible symptoms in 48–72 hours but changes may be irreversible after exposure for many days. The rate of development of the pulmonary reaction is influenced by a number of metabolic and pharmacological factors as well as by the inspired concentration. Prolonged exposure to concentrations in excess of 50 per cent appears to be necessary. Interruption of the exposure by periods breathing lower concentrations appears to have a protective effect. In practice uninterrupted administration of really high concentrations of oxygen is mainly confined to patients with tracheostomies or endotracheal tubes who are receiving artificial ventilation. Clinically overt oxygen toxicity is almost unheard of as a consequence of oxygen administration using conventional masks. Whenever patients require high concentrations of oxygen, care must be taken to ensure that the inspired level is maintained at the lowest compatible with a safe arterial oxygen tension. Once the condition is established, no treatment other than lowering of the oxygen concentration is of any avail—and this may be impossible.

5. FIRE
The hazard of fire should not be underestimated. Many materials which are

normally relatively non-flammable burn furiously in an oxygen-rich atmosphere. Naked flames and smoking must be absolutely forbidden in the vicinity of oxygen administration.

Domiciliary oxygen therapy

There are a few instances in which oxygen therapy may be valuable at home.

1. TO AID EXERCISE IN THE HOME

Oxygen therapy can be used, for example, when climbing stairs, washing, or moving from room to room. The cylinder should be situated strategically and long lengths of low-pressure plastic tubing used to make oxygen available at a distance.

2. PORTABLE OXYGEN

In a few patients exercise is much extended by use of oxygen and they may find it useful out of doors. It is very desirable to test a patient's response to oxygen under controlled conditions before supplying portable equipment. Detailed instruction is required.

3. LONG-TERM OXYGEN THERAPY

It has been suggested that long-term administration of oxygen may benefit patients in chronic ventilatory failure secondary to chronic bronchitis. The effect of breathing low concentrations of oxygen for up to 15 hours a day (mainly at night) is being investigated in a number of centres but it is not yet sufficiently tried to be recommended for general use.

4. PLACEBO EFFECT

All oxygen administration exerts a strong placebo effect. Where advanced disease is causing great anguish the availability of oxygen may do much to relieve the worst moments even if its use seems illogical. The hazards of inappropriate use may sometimes be acceptable under these circumstances.

Note

Domiciliary oxygen therapy requires that at least one member of the household be sufficiently fit and practically minded to change valves and turn cylinders on and off. This takes considerable effort and hypoxic patients are seldom able or inclined to make the necessary effort themselves.

APPENDIX: SI UNITS OF PRESSURE

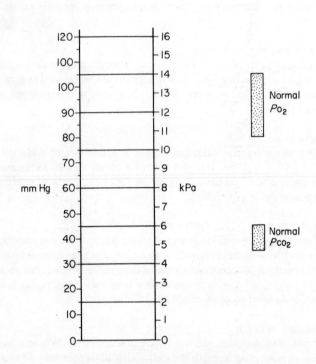

Nomogram relating mmHg and kPa
Even numbers of kPa relate exactly to convenient values of mmHg at
intervals of 15 mmHg and some of these values may be worth remembering.
$$1 \text{ kPa} = 7.5 \text{ mmHg}$$
$$1 \text{ mmHg} = 0.13 \text{ kPa}$$

FURTHER READING

The student in search of further information on a particular clinical subject is advised to refer to:
CROFTON J. & DOUGLAS A. (1975) *Respiratory Diseases*, 2nd edition. Oxford, Blackwell Scientific Publications.
This excellent reference work will usually provide him with what he requires or direct him to suitable source references. The following annotated list suggests some other works which will repay exploration.

Respiratory physiology and pulmonary function tests

BATES D.V. & CHRISTIE R.V. (1964) *Respiratory Function in Disease*. Philadelphia, Saunders.
(Notable for worked examples correlating clinical and physiological findings.)

CAMPBELL E.J.M., AGOSTONI E. & NEWSOM DAVIS J. (1970) *The Respiratory Muscles*. London, Lloyd-Luke.
(Excellent review of lung mechanics and comprehensive review of ventilatory control.)

COMROE J.H. Jr, FORSTER R.E., DUBOIS A.B., BRISCOE W.A. & CARLSEN E. (1962) *The Lung*. Chicago, Year Book Medical Publishers.
(Basic text on pulmonary physiology and function testing; good diagrams.)

COTES J.E. (1975) *Lung Function*, 3rd edition. Oxford, Blackwell Scientific Publications.
(Essential reference work on background to pulmonary function testing.)

CUMMING G. & SEMPLE S.G. (1973) *Disorders of the Respiratory System*. Oxford, Blackwell Scientific Publications.
(First 155 pages; Gas transport and control of ventilation particularly well done.)

FENN W.O. & RAHN H. (eds) (1964) *Handbook of Physiology, Section 3, Respiration*, Vols 1 and 2. Washington, American Physiological Society.
(Monumental reference work; very valuable despite age.)

NUNN J.F. (1969) *Applied Respiratory Physiology, with Special Reference to Anaesthesia*. London, Butterworth.
(Clear and comprehensive.)

WEST J.B. (1976) *Ventilation/Blood-flow and Gas Exchange*, 3rd edition. Oxford, Blackwell Scientific Publications.
(Readable essay with exposition of O_2–CO_2 diagram.)

WEST J.B. (1974) *Respiratory Physiology—the Essentials*. Oxford, Blackwell Scientific Publications.
(Concise, clear and inexpensive.)

Radiology

SIMON G. (1962) *Principles of Chest X-ray Diagnosis*, 2nd edition. London, Butterworth.
(Informative, systematic approach.)
SQUIRE L.F., COLIACE W.M. & STRUTYNSKY N. (1970) *Exercises in Diagnostic Radiology, I: The Chest*. Philadelphia, Saunders.
(Well illustrated, stimulating question and answer format.)

Respiratory infections

GARROD L.P., LAMBERT H.P. & O'GRADY F. (1973) *Antibiotic and Chemotherapy*. Edinburgh, Churchill Livingstone.
(First part; review of the antibiotics; second part: their application in disease.)
KNIGHT V. (1973) *Viral and Mycoplasmal Infection of the Respiratory Tract*. Philadelphia, Lea and Febiger.
(Thorough, systematic, many references.)

Asthma

AUSTEN K.F. & LICHTENSTEIN L.M. (eds) (1973) *Asthma, Physiology, Immunopharmacology and Treatment*. New York, Academic Press.
(Excellent up-to-date review of underlying mechanisms.)
CIBA FOUNDATION GUEST SYMPOSIUM (1971) *Identification of Asthma*. Edinburgh, Churchill Livingstone.
(Useful review of the problem of definition and of pathogenesis.)

Fibrosing alveolitis

LIVINGSTONE J.L., LEWIS J.G., REID L. & JEFFERSON K. (1964) Diffuse interstitial pulmonary fibrosis, *Quart. J. Med.*, 33, 71.
(Very informative account of large series.)
TURNER-WARWICK M. (1972) Cryptogenic fibrosing alveolitis, *Brit. J. Hosp. Med.*, 7, 697.
(Includes discussion of relationship to other conditions.)

Sarcoidosis

SCADDING J.G. (1967) *Sarcoidosis*. London, Eyre and Spottiswoode.
(Definitive reference work.)

Chronic bronchitis, airways obstruction and emphysema

CUMMING G. & HUNT L.B. (eds) (1968) *Form and Function in the Human Lung*. Edinburgh, Livingstone.
(Symposium centred upon chronic airways obstruction and emphysema.)

FILLEY G.F. (1967) *Pulmonary Insufficiency and Respiratory Failure*. Philadelphia, Lea and Febiger.
(Lucid, readable account.)

HEARD B.E. (1969) *Pathology of Chronic Bronchitis and Emphysema*. London, Churchill.
(Beautiful account of pathology; worth looking at if only for illustrations.)

MAY J.R. (1968) *Chemotherapy of Chronic Bronchitis*. London, English Universities Press.
(Valuable, well-summarised conclusions.)

ROYAL COLLEGE OF PHYSICIANS (1971) *Smoking and Health Now*. London, Pitman Medical.
(Useful assimilation of evidence.)

SYKES M.K., MCNICHOL M.W. & CAMPBELL R.J.M. (1976) *Respiratory Failure*, 2nd edition, Oxford, Blackwell Scientific Publications.
(Physiological and practical aspects clearly dealt with.)

Carcinoma of the Bronchus

DEELEY T.J. (ed.) (1971) *Carcinoma of the Bronchus*. London, Butterworth.
(Comprehensive account; emphasis on radiotherapy.)

ROYAL COLLEGE OF PHYSICIANS (1971) *Smoking and Health Now*. London, Pitman Medical.

STRADLING P. (1973) *Diagnostic Bronchoscopy*, 2nd edition, London, Livingstone. (Worth looking at if only for illustrations.)

Occupational lung disease

MUIR D.C.F. (ed.) (1972) *Clinical Aspects of Inhaled Particles*. London, Heinemann.
(Useful sections on deposition and clearance, also asbestos-induced diseases.)

PARKES W.R. (1974) *Occupational Lung Disorders*. London, Butterworth.
(Definitive reference work.)

Oxygen therapy

SYKES M.K., MCNICHOL M.W. & CAMPBELL E.J.M. (1976) *Respiratory Failure*. 2nd edition, Oxford, Blackwell Scientific Publications.
GREEN I.D. (1967) Choice of method for administration of oxygen, *Brit. med. J.* 3, 593.
(Informative assessment of performance of different masks.)

INDEX